sports nutrition for
YOUNG ATHLETES

Anita Bean

FIREFLY BOOKS

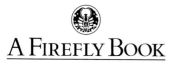

A FIREFLY BOOK

Published by Firefly Books Ltd. 2012

First printing

Publisher Cataloging-in-Publication Data (U.S.)

Bean, Anita.
    Sports nutrition for young athletes / Anita Bean.
[160] p. : col. photos. ; cm.
Includes bibliographical references and index.
Summary: Details best sports nutrition for young athletes, including meal plans, recipes and discussion of body mass index.
ISBN-13: 978-1-77085-030-9 (pbk.)
1. Teenage athletes — Nutrition. 2. Child athletes — Nutrition.
3. Nutrition — . I. Title.
613.2083 dc23   RJ206.B346 2010

Library and Archives Canada Cataloguing in Publication

Bean, Anita
    Sports nutrition for young athletes / Anita Bean.
Includes bibliographical references and index.
ISBN 978-1-77085-030-9
    1. Teenage athletes—Nutrition. 2. Child athletes—Nutrition.
I. Title.
RJ206.B39 2012   613.2083   C2011-907757-4

Published in the United States by
Firefly Books (U.S.) Inc.
P.O. Box 1338, Ellicott Station
Buffalo, New York 14205

Published in Canada by
Firefly Books Ltd.
66 Leek Crescent
Richmond Hill, Ontario L4B 1H1

Printed and bound in Spain by GraphyCems

This title was developed by
A & C Black Publishers Ltd
36 Soho Square, London
W1D 3QY
Designed by James Watson
Commissioned by Charlotte Croft
Edited by Kate Turvey

Photo credits:
Cover photograph © Shutterstock (back); © Getty Images (front, top); © Bananastock Ltd (front, bottom)
Inside photographs © Shutterstock 10, 12, 14, 40, 46, 51, 68, 73, 82, 84, 86, 92, 95, 98, 101, 102, 114, 122, 132, 136, 141; istock 2, 23, 43, 49, 64, 106; Punchstock 15, 18, 57, 72; Comstock 56, 107; Anita Bean v; A&C Black vii

CONTENTS

ACKNOWLEDGMENTS

I would like to thank my daughters, Chloe and Lucy (pictured below), who have been the inspiration for writing this book. They are both competitive swimmers who fit a demanding daily training and eating schedule around their school and social life! I am immensely proud of their achievements. I must also thank my husband Simon, without whose support, patience and energy this book would not have been possible.

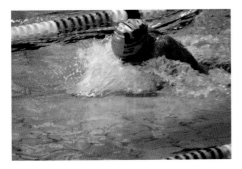 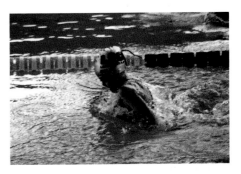

INTRODUCTION

I have been advising coaches and parents of young athletes as well as young athletes themselves (including my own children) for many years and am delighted to have this opportunity to share my knowledge and experience.

There's no doubt that what children eat affects their health as well as their performance in sport. If they eat a poor quality diet then they not only risk illness but they will not be able to train and compete to the best of their ability. But if they eat a healthy diet that provides the correct amount of energy and nutrients, then they will enjoy better health and improved performance in their sport.

The nutritional requirements of young athletes are not too dissimilar from those of non-athletes but there are a number of special considerations. The most obvious one is meeting their energy needs, which not only have to support growth and development but also their level of activity. Young athletes exercising for an hour a day may need an extra 400–500 kcal; those training for two hours or more daily may require an extra 1000 kcal. They also need proportionally more carbohydrate, more protein and more vitamins and minerals. Chapter 1, The nutritional needs of young athletes, provides practical guidance on how to plan a healthy diet for sport.

As well as ensuring they get enough fuel and are eating the right types of food, young athletes also have to consider the timing of their food and drink intake before, during and after each training session. Chapter 2, Eating for sport, explains the optimal timing of meals, snacks and drinks as well as menu suggestions.

There may also be concerns about body weight and body composition. These issues need to be treated sensitively and it is important that young athletes seek correct advice before embarking on any regime. Chapter 3, Weight and sports performance, provides sensible weight loss and weight gain strategies to help you plan their program.

Many young athletes take supplements, such as sports drinks, vitamins and protein supplements. But often they do not know exactly what they are or how they work. In Chapter 4 I consider the evidence for the most popular supplements and tell you which ones (may) work and which ones don't.

What young athletes eat and drink in the weeks and days before a competition, as well as on the day of the competition, will make a big difference to their performance. So it's important that they have a nutrition strategy to give them the competitive edge. Chapter 5 will help you devise one.

To help you put the nutrition information into practice I have devised simple and tasty recipes for main meals, vegetarian meals, soups, desserts and baking at the end of this book. Hopefully, these will inspire you and your young athletes to get in the kitchen and get cooking!

It's not essential that young athletes eat a perfect diet all the time, but provided they get it right about 80 percent of the time, then they will have a great chance of putting in their best performance.

I hope you find this book helpful.

Anita Bean
June 2010

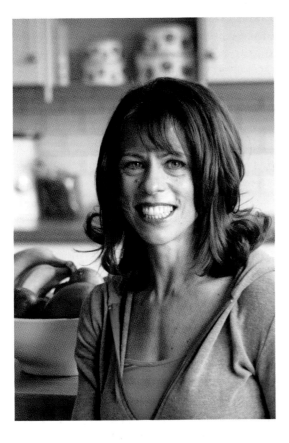

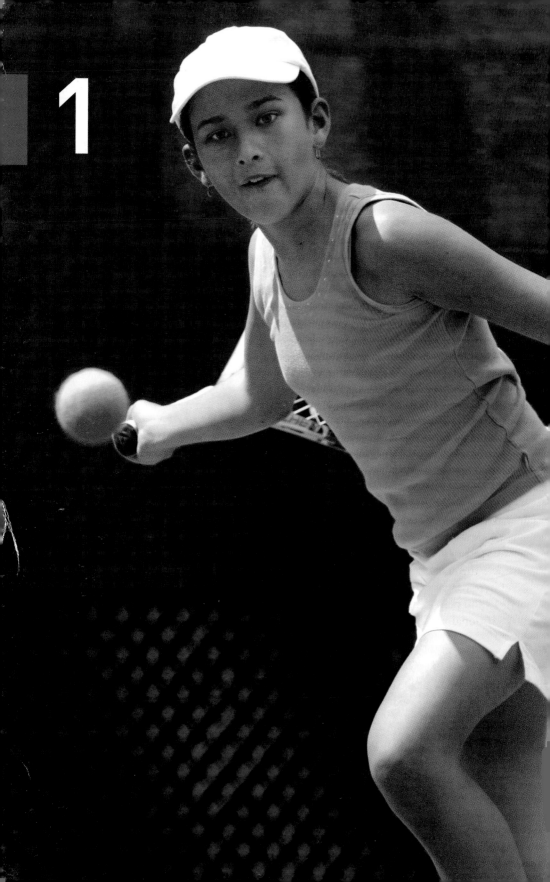

1

THE NUTRITIONAL NEEDS OF YOUNG ATHLETES

How can good nutritional practices help young athletes perform better? According to the International Olympic Committee (IOC) in its 2003 Consensus statement:

> The amount, composition and timing of food intake can profoundly affect sports performance. Good nutritional practice will help athletes train hard, recover quickly and adapt more effectively with less risk of illness and injury. Athletes should adopt specific nutritional strategies before and during competition to help maximize their performance.

What this means, in practice, is that a healthy diet will help young athletes:

- have more energy for training;
- increase their stamina and strength;
- recover faster;
- reduce their chances of illness and minor injuries;
- gain a competitive edge.

During childhood and adolescence, growth and development is rapid, and this places high energy and nutritional demands on the young athlete's body. Clearly, their diet needs to provide enough energy, carbohydrate, fat, protein, vitamins and minerals to fuel growth as well as training and recovery. The energy and nutrient requirements for boys and girls aged 4–18 years are shown in Tables 1.1 and 1.2. These values should cover the needs of 95 percent of children. But there are no specific values for athletic children, who will almost certainly need to eat more than their non-active peers. To help you plan their food intake, this chapter provides a basic guide to young athletes' nutritional needs.

Table 1.1 Dietary reference values for boys aged 4–18

	Dietary reference value (DRV)	4–6 years	7–10 years	11–14 years	15–18 years
Energy	Estimated average requirement (EAR)	1715 kcal	1979 kcal	2220 kcal	2755 kcal
Fat	Max. 35% energy	67 g	77 g	86 g	107 g
Saturated fat	Max. 11% energy	21 g	24 g	27 g	34 g
Carbohydrate	Min. 50% energy	229 g	263 g	296 g	367 g
Added sugars*	Max. 11% energy	50 g	58 g	65 g	81 g
Fiber**	8 g per 1000 kcal	14 g	16 g	18 g	22 g
Protein		19.7 g	28 g	42 g	55 g
Iron		6.1 mg	8.7 mg	11.3 mg	11.3 mg
Zinc		6.5 mg	7.0 mg	9.0 mg	9.5 mg
Calcium		450 mg	550 mg	1000 mg	1000 mg
Vitamin A		500 mcg	500 mcg	600 mcg	700 mcg
Vitamin C		30 mg	30 mg	35 mg	40 mg
Folate		100 mcg	150 mcg	200 mcg	200 mcg
Salt***		3 g	5 g	6 g	6 g

Source: Department of Health (1991)

Notes
* Non-milk extrinsic sugars
** Proportion of adult DRV (18 g), i.e. 8 g/1000 kcal
*** Scientific Advisory Committee on Nutrition (2003)

Table 1.2 Dietary reference values for girls aged 4–18

	Dietary reference value (DRV)	4–6 years	7–10 years	11–14 years	15–18 years
Energy	Estimated average requirement (EAR)	1545 kcal	1740 kcal	1845 kcal	2110 kcal
Fat	Max. 35% energy	60 g	68 g	72 g	82 g
Saturated fat	Max. 11% energy	19 g	21 g	23 g	26 g
Carbohydrate	Min. 50% energy	206 g	232 g	246 g	281 g
Added sugars*	Max. 11% energy	45 g	51 g	54 g	62 g
Fiber**	8 g per 1000 kcal	12 g	14 g	15 g	17 g
Protein		19.7 g	28 g	41 g	45 g
Iron		6.1 mg	8.7 mg	14.8 mg	14.8 mg
Zinc		6.5 mg	7.0 mg	9.0 mg	7.0 mg
Calcium		450 mg	550 mg	800 mg	800 mg
Vitamin A		500 mcg	500 mcg	600 mcg	600 mcg
Vitamin C		30 mg	30 mg	35 mg	40 mg
Folate		100 mcg	150 mcg	200 mcg	200 mcg
Salt***		3 g	5 g	6 g	6 g

Source: Department of Health (1991)

Notes
* Non-milk extrinsic sugars
** Proportion of adult DRV (18 g), i.e. 8 g/1000 kcal
*** Scientific Advisory Committee on Nutrition (2003)

ENERGY, CALORIES – WHAT'S THE DIFFERENCE?

Most people think of energy as good, calories bad. In fact, they refer to the same thing! Calories are a measure of energy, whether it's the energy content of food or the energy cost of exercise. When we talk about calories in the everyday sense, we actually mean kilocalories (1000 calories = 1 kilocalorie or 1 kcal). This is what you'll see on the nutrition information panel on food labels and physical activity charts.

WHAT IS THE PHYSICAL ACTIVITY LEVEL (PAL)?

The PAL is the total energy cost of a person's physical activity throughout the day, expressed as a ratio of their basal metabolic rate (BMR). The more active they are, the higher the PAL. Most young athletes would probably have a PAL of 2.0. Table 1.3 describes a range of PALs.

Table 1.3 Physical activity level (PAL)

Physical activity level (PAL)	Description	Examples
1.4	Sedentary	Mainly sitting
1.5	Sedentary – moderately active	Mainly sitting/a little physical activity
1.6	Moderately active	Some walking/moderate activity
1.8	Active	Daily moderate activity
2.0	Very active	Daily intense activity or sport

How much energy do young athletes need?

The amount of energy (or calories) young athletes need to consume depends on several things: their age, their weight, how much muscle they have and how active they are. In general, the heavier they are, the more muscle they have; and the more active they are, the greater their daily expenditure, therefore the more energy they need to consume. In addition, they need an extra 60 to 100 kcal per day for growth (Department of Health, 1991).

Table 1.4 gives the estimated energy needs for 10–17 year olds for different body weights and physical activity levels (PALs). The BMR (*see* the box, "What is the basal metabolic rate (BMR)?") is derived from a formula based on body weight (Schofield *et al.*, 1985).

As you can see from Table 1.4, young athletes (assuming a PAL of 2.0) have considerably higher energy needs than their non-athletic peers. For example, an athletic 65 kg boy (PAL 2.0) would need about 3612 kcal a day, while a 60 kg girl (PAL 2.0) would need 2990 kcal – almost an extra 900 kcal compared with non-athletic teenagers with the same body weight (PAL 1.4–1.5).

Unfortunately, there are no published data on the energy cost of various activities for children, but it is possible to make an estimate by extrapolating from adult values. Table 1.5 provides values for adults with different body weights, and should give you a rough idea of how much energy young athletes burn during training. Bear in mind, though, that these values may underestimate the actual energy burn for younger children. Younger children use more energy per kg body weight than do teenagers and adults (Macdougall *et al.*, 1982). Generally, the younger the child the higher the relative energy cost. A 7 year old, for example, would burn 25–30 percent more energy per kg body weight than would an adult walking or running at the same speed. This is explained by the relative "wastefulness" of energy in children, due to lack of coordination. As their proficiency improves, though, the energy cost decreases. As a rule of thumb, for children 8–10 years old, add 20–25 percent to the adult values; add 10–15 percent for children aged 11–14 years.

WHAT IS THE BASAL METABOLIC RATE (BMR)?

At least 60 percent of a person's daily energy burn is used to keep the heart beating, the organs functioning and the core body temperature stable. This is called the basal metabolic rate (BMR), and is higher for children and teenagers than for adults.

Table 1.4 Estimated average energy requirements of children and adolescents according to body weight and physical activity level

Weight (kg)	BMR kcal/d	PAL				
		1.4	**1.5**	**1.6**	**1.8**	**2.0**
Boys						
30	1189	1675	1794	1914	2153	2368
35	1278	1794	1914	2057	2297	2559
40	1366	1914	2057	2177	2464	2727
45	1455	2033	2177	2320	2632	2919
50	1543	2153	2321	2464	2775	3086
55	1632	2297	2440	2608	2943	3253
60	1720	2416	2584	2751	3086	3445
65	1809	2536	2703	2895	3254	3612
Girls						
30	1095	1531	1651	1746	1962	2201
35	1163	1627	1715	1866	2081	2321
40	1229	1722	1842	1962	2201	2464
45	1297	1818	1938	2081	2344	2584
50	1364	1913	2033	2177	2464	2727
55	1430	2009	2153	2297	2584	2871
60	1498	2105	2249	2392	2703	2990

Source: Department of Health (1991)

Table 1.5 The energy cost of various activities

Body weight (kg)	44	50	56	62	68	74
Body weight (lb)	97	110	123	137	159	163
Badminton	265	300	325	360	395	430
Basketball	365	415	460	510	565	610
Competitive	390	445	500	550	600	655
Boxing	400	455	510	565	620	675
Circuit training	350	380	410	440	470	500
Cycling @ 12 mph	360	390	425	460	495	530
Racing	450	510	570	630	690	750
Dancing	270	295	320	345	370	395
Hockey	360	405	450	500	545	590
Football	355	400	445	490	535	580
Horse riding	240	275	310	345	370	405
Rowing	600	660	720	780	830	890
Running @ 6.5 mph	425	480	535	590	650	705
@ 10 mph	620	690	765	835	900	965
Squash	515	580	645	710	785	850
Swimming: slow	230	260	290	320	350	380
Fast laps	400	445	490	535	580	625
Tennis	300	340	375	415	455	490
Weight training	350	395	440	485	530	575
Walking 5 mph	200	220	240	260	280	300

What are the best fuels for exercise?

Muscles burn a mixture of carbohydrate, fat and (to a much smaller extent) protein during exercise. The amounts and proportions of each fuel burned will depend on the intensity and duration of the activity.

As a rule of thumb, the higher the training intensity, the higher the proportion of carbohydrate used. During high-intensity aerobic activities, such as fast running or fast swimming, the muscles burn mostly carbohydrate and proportionally less fat.

During lower-intensity activities, such as jogging or slow swimming, the muscles burn fewer calories per minute and proportionally less carbohydrate.

Most of the carbohydrate is supplied by the muscles' store of glycogen. But this store is relatively small – enough to fuel perhaps 1½–2 hours of intense exercise. Once glycogen levels become depleted, exercise starts to feel much harder and fatigue sets in. Starting a training session with high levels of muscle glycogen will help delay fatigue and increase endurance.

Think of filling up a car with gas before setting off on a journey. If you start with a full fuel tank, you will be able to travel further; if you start with low fuel levels you won't be able to travel as far. Similarly, for athletes, if they begin training with high glycogen levels they will be able to train harder and longer before reaching fatigue point. If they begin training with low glycogen levels, they will tire more easily and perform below their potential. To delay fatigue, encourage young athletes to eat a carbohydrate-rich diet during the 24–48 hours before training.

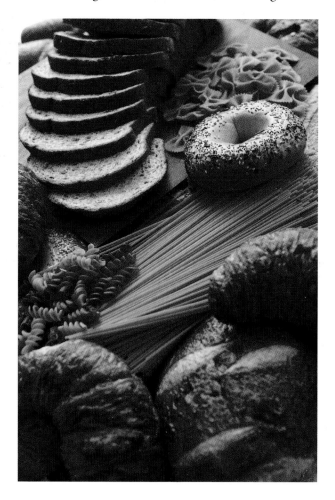

How much carbohydrate should young athletes eat each day?

This will depend on their weight – or, more accurately, the amount of muscle they are carrying – and how active they are each day. The heavier they are and the more active they are, the more carbohydrate they should eat. Table 1.6 gives the estimated carbohydrate requirements for athletes with different body weights for various activity levels. Young athletes training for up to 2 hours a day would need around 5–7 g carbohydrate for each 1 kg body weight; those training for more than 2 hours, would need 7–10 g/kg body weight/day. For example, a 60 kg athlete training for 1–2 hours each day would need 360–420 g carbohydrate daily, or 420–600 g daily if training for 2–4 hours.

Table 1.6 Carbohydrate needs for young athletes

Number of hours' exercise per day	Carbohydrate/kg body weight/day	Carbohydrate/day for a 50 kg person	Carbohydrate/day for a 60 kg person	Carbohydrate/day for a 70 kg person
0–1	5–6 g	250–300 g	300–360 g	350–420 g
1–2	6–7 g	300–350 g	360–420 g	420–490 g
3–4	7–8 g	350–400 g	420–480 g	490–560 g
4+	8–10 g	400–500 g	480–600 g	560–700 g

Tell me how to do it!

To give you an idea of how much food an athlete would need to eat, the following menu contains approximately 400 g carbohydrate – enough to fuel around 2 hours' daily exercise for someone weighing 60 kg.

Sample menu
Breakfast
2 slices of toast with margarine and honey
2 bananas

Lunch
1 large baked potato with margarine, half a can of baked beans and 2 tablespoons (40 g) grated cheese
Salad
1 fruit yogurt

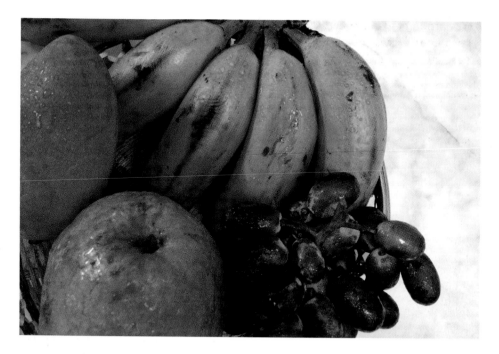

Dinner
Large bowl of pasta (125 g dry weight)
Chicken breast (200g) or cheese (40g)
Vegetables

Snacks
2 pieces of fresh fruit
400 ml fruit juice
2 granola bars
1 fruit yogurt

Energy
2800 kcal

Carbohydrate
411 g

As a rule of thumb, young athletes should be able to meet their carbohydrate requirements by eating:

- 4–6 portions of grains/potatoes;
- 5 portions of fruit/vegetables;
- 2–4 portions of dairy products.

One portion of grains/potatoes is equivalent to two slices of bread or 150 g potatoes; a portion of fruit is equivalent to a banana, and a portion of dairy is equivalent to a glass (200 ml) of milk (*see* page 37).

Table 1.7 will help you work out how much food a young athlete should eat, as will checking the carbohydrate values on food labels.

Table 1.7 The carbohydrate content of different foods

Food	Energy (kcal)	Carbohydrate (g)
Apples (one, 100 g)	47	12
Baked beans (200 g)	162	30
Bananas (one, 100 g)	95	23
Cookies (one, 15 g)	70	10
Bran flakes (40 g)	132	29
Bread (one slice, 35 g)	80	15
Cereal bar (one, 30 g)	140	18
Pancake (one, 70 g)	345	44
Jam or honey (15 g)	40	10
Milk, partly-skimmed (300 ml)	138	14
Oatcakes (one, 13 g)	54	8
Orange juice (200 ml)	72	18
Pasta (85 g dry weight)	196	64
Pita bread (one, 60 g)	160	34
Oatmeal (200 g)	166	23
Potatoes (200 g)	150	34
Rice (85 g dried weight)	303	69
Roll (one, 50 g)	120	22
Shreddies (40 g)	138	31
Corn (80 g)	89	16
Weetabix (two, 40 g)	141	30
Yogurt (one container, 150 g)	117	21

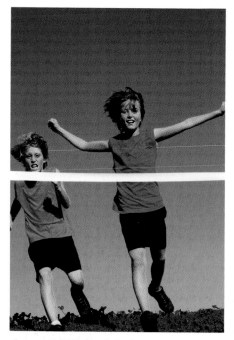

How can I tell whether they are eating enough – or too much?

It can be tricky to judge exactly how much food young athletes should eat. In an ideal world, everyone would be guided by their appetite, and eat just the right amount of food to maintain their body weight and fuel their activities. But, in practice, it's not always easy to get it right! As a rough guide, if young athletes always seem hungry, struggle to recover fully between training sessions, and frequently lack energy while training, this suggests that they may need to step up their energy and carbohydrate intake.

Other signs that they may not be consuming enough energy and carbohydrate include frequent colds, infections and minor illnesses. This is because a suboptimal intake of carbohydrate can reduce the availability of fuel to the immune cells and increase the production of stress hormones (adrenaline and cortisol), which reduces immune function. All this makes a person more susceptible to infection and illness.

On the other hand, if young athletes are putting on unwanted pounds, cutting back on carbohydrates – as well as fat – will help them lose weight. The body can store only around 400–500 g glycogen; any excess carbohydrate is converted to fat. The best way to prevent weight gain is to keep a check on portion sizes and divide their daily carbohydrate intake into several moderate-sized meals or snacks throughout the day. Make sure they don't eat all their carbohydrate in one big meal. And, if they have a tendency to gain weight easily, they should avoid snacking on "energy dense" carbohydrate foods such as cookies, chips, candy and chocolate.

Which are the best carbs to eat?

The best foods to eat for performance are those that contain carbohydrate along with high levels of fiber and other nutrients, such as vitamins and minerals. Encourage young athletes to opt for whole grains rather than refined versions: wholemeal bread instead of white bread; wholegrain pasta instead of ordinary pasta; wholegrain rice instead of white; and wholegrain breakfast cereals such as oatmeal, whole-wheat cereals, rice cakes and muesli. They should also include lots of starchy vegetables, such as potatoes, sweet potatoes and corn; as well as legumes (beans and lentils), which provide protein as well as carbohydrate. Nutritious snack choices include fresh and dried fruit – these foods contain natural sugars as well as all-important vitamins, minerals, antioxidants and fiber.

All of these foods will provide young athletes with sustained energy. Their high fiber content means that they digest and break down more slowly than high-sugar foods (e.g. sweets, carbonated drinks) and refined starchy foods made from white flour (e.g. white bread). This means that they are digested more slowly and release glucose into the bloodstream over a longer period. Eating them with protein, such as fish, cheese or milk, would produce an even more gradual energy release. So, eating breakfast cereal with milk, potato with tuna, or bread with cheese, will fuel the body for longer.

CARBOHYDRATE-RICH FOODS AT A GLANCE

Good main meal choices	Good snack choices	Choose less often
Wholegrain pasta	Fresh fruit, e.g. apples,	White bread and rolls,
Wholegrain rice	pears, oranges,	French bread and
Baked or boiled	peaches, apricots,	bagels
potatoes	bananas, grapes, kiwi	White rice
Sweet potatoes	fruit, strawberries,	High-sugar breakfast
Corn	mango	cereals
Wholegrain bread, rolls,	Dried fruit, e.g. raisins,	
pita, wraps	apricots, figs	
Wholegrain breakfast	Rice cakes	
cereals	Oat cakes	
Oatmeal	Wholegrain crackers	
Beans, chickpeas, lentils	Cereal bars	
	Crumpets	
	Plain popcorn	

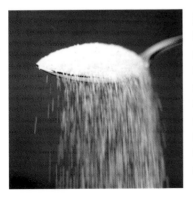

Is sugar good or bad for young athletes?

Sugar is a carbohydrate, which means it is an energy source for the body. Like starch, it can be used to fuel exercise, convert into glycogen or turn into fat. It is absorbed rapidly into the bloodstream, which can be useful during long, intense training sessions when the muscles may run low on glycogen and need extra fuel quickly. Consuming sugar (for example, a sports drink, a cereal bar or dried fruit) would be beneficial for performance when exercising hard for longer than an hour, but unnecessary for shorter sessions (*see* Chapter 2, page 45). Sugar-containing drinks and foods may also be beneficial for refueling muscles during the two-hour period after exercise (*see* Chapter 2, page 54).

However, there are many myths when it comes to sugar and performance. For example, many people believe that consuming high-sugar foods or drinks will give them extra energy for exercise. I frequently see young athletes munching sweets and chocolate bars on their way to training sessions, or swigging sugary drinks just before setting out. In fact, researchers have shown that the opposite holds true – consuming sugar before exercise, does *not* improve performance or stamina (Burke *et al.*, 1998; Wu and Williams, 2006). The problem is that eating lots of sugar triggers high levels of insulin in the bloodstream, which transports sugar out of the bloodstream rapidly, leaving the athlete with less available energy. This rebound effect can make athletes feel tired, weak and light-headed. Instead, encourage them to eat a healthy meal based on potatoes, wholegrain bread or pasta two to four hours before training, or a snack based on fruit or cereals 30 minutes before exercise (*see* Chapter 2, page 43–44).

Remember that sugar is harmful for teeth and lacks other useful nutrients, so young athletes should keep it to a minimum in their day-to-day diet, particularly between meals when they can do the most damage to the teeth. If they must have a sweet treat, it is better that they consume sugar at mealtimes when it is less likely to cause decay. Sugary drinks and sports drinks are highly acidic and can, over time, cause a thinning of the enamel and a change in the texture, shape and appearance of teeth. Minimize the risk of acid erosion by getting young athletes to use a drinks bottle with a spout, direct the drink towards the back of the mouth and, ideally, have some water afterwards to wash away the acid and sugar.

Sugar that occurs naturally in foods such as fruit, vegetables and milk is locked in to the structure of the food and tends to be less harmful to the teeth. These foods supply lots of other nutrients, so are a healthier choice.

How much sugar should young athletes eat?

There are no official dietary guidelines (although this is currently under review at the time of going to print) but the guideline daily amount (GDA) for "added" (or "non-milk extrinsic sugars," NME) sugars is 11 percent of the daily energy intake. However, food labels do not distinguish between "added" and "natural" sugars (such as those found in fruit and milk), and give you the "total sugar" sugar content of the product. The GDA for total sugar is 20 percent of daily energy. Table 1.8 shows the GDA for different ages. These values apply to non-athletic children. As athletic children have higher energy needs they can consume a little more sugar, although this should still be within 20 percent of daily energy intake.

Table 1.8 Guideline daily amounts for sugar

	11–14 years	15–18 years
Girls		
Total sugars	90 g	105 g
NME sugars	50 g	60 g
Boys		
Total sugars	110 g	140 g
NME sugars	60 g	75 g

Check food labels for sugar. Foods containing more than 15 g sugar per 100 g, or drinks containing more than 7.5 g sugar per 100 ml, are high in sugar, and should be kept to a minimum.

SUGAR GUIDE FOR ATHLETES

- Young athletes should save their sugar for exercise. During training sessions lasting more than an hour, diluted fruit juice and sports drinks, dried fruit and cereal bars will help fuel tiring muscles and improve endurance.
- At other times, if they want something sweet, they should opt for foods that contain additional nutrients: fresh fruit, dried fruit, fruit yogurt, fruit juice, smoothies, granola bars and breakfast cereal.
- Set a sensible daily limit of two or three portions for high-sugar foods – e.g. candy, chocolate, cookies, cakes and puddings (*see* pages 35–36).
- They should drink water after eating or drinking anything sugary, to help wash the sugar away, or chew gum to stimulate the production of saliva, which can neutralize the acid.

How much protein do young athletes need?

Their diet needs to cover their protein requirements for growth and development, for day-to-day repair and maintenance of body proteins, as well as a little extra for fueling intense exercise. Non-athletic children aged 13–18 years need around 0.85–1 g protein for each 1 kg of body weight, or about 55 g for someone weighing 60 kg (Department of Health, 1991). There are no published values for young athletes – only for adult athletes – but it is estimated that they need more than non-athletes, around 1.2 to 1.4 g per 1 kg body weight – that's 72–84 g for someone weighing 60 kg (Boisseau *et al.*, 2007). Adult athletes require a similar amount, between 1.2 and

1.7 g protein/kg body weight (IAAF, 2007). This goes to repair the muscle proteins broken down during intense exercise, and also to make new muscle tissue.

The protein needs for young athletes of different body weights are given in Table 1.9.

Table 1.9 Protein needs of young athletes

Body weight	Daily protein requirement
44 kg (97 lb)	53–62 g
50 kg (110 lb)	60–70 g
56 kg (123 lb)	67–78 g
62 kg (137 kg)	74–87 g
68 kg (159 lb)	82–95 g

What are the best ways to get protein?

Protein is found in many foods. The richest sources include lean meat such as chicken and turkey, fish, eggs, cheese, milk, yogurt, beans, lentils, nuts, soya and Quorn (a mycoprotein). Other useful sources include cereal-based foods, such as bread, pasta and breakfast cereals. Including two to three portions of protein-rich foods daily makes it relatively easy for young athletes to meet their daily requirement. You can work out the protein content of a young athlete's diet by checking Table 1.10, as well as the nutrition information on food labels.

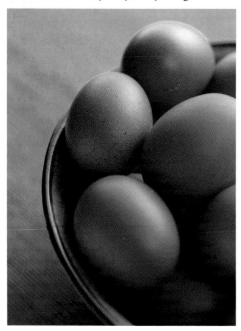

Table 1.10 The protein content of different foods

Food	Protein (g)
Baked beans (one small tin, 200 g)	10
Bread (two slices, 70 g)	6
Cheese (one matchbox-sized piece, 40 g)	10
Chicken (one breast, 125 g)	30
Eggs (one)	8
Lentils (three tablespoons, 120 g)	9
Milk (one glass, 200 ml)	7
Pasta (230 g cooked)	7
Peanut butter (one teaspoon, 20 g)	5
Peanuts (50 g)	12
Quorn burger (one, 50 g)	6
Red kidney beans (three tablespoons, 120 g)	10
Salmon (one filet, 150 g)	30
Steak (one lean filet, 105 g)	31
Tofu burger (one, 60 g)	5
Tuna (one small tin, 100 g)	24
Turkey (one breast, 125 g)	31
Yogurt (one container, 150 g)	6

Can eating too little or too much protein be harmful?

Eating too little protein every now and then isn't a problem because the body is able to adapt to different intakes. If dietary supplies dip, the body tries to conserve existing protein by recycling old proteins into new ones and excreting less protein. In other words, it becomes more efficient in conserving protein.

However, if young athletes eat very little protein for weeks – cutting out meat, fish, dairy products and legumes – then they may develop symptoms of protein deficiency: wasting and shrinkage of muscle tissue, edema (build-up of fluids, particularly in the feet and ankles), anemia and slow growth. This condition is very rare, however, even among vegetarians and vegans.

Eating too much protein is unlikely to be a problem either. Any protein not needed for repairing and making muscle tissue is broken down by the body into other compounds (such as urea) and excreted in the urine. However, this may place extra stress on the liver and kidneys, so you should try to stick to the protein guidelines above.

Will extra protein make young athletes stronger?

It's tempting to think that a high intake of protein – whether from food or supplements – will build bigger and stronger muscles. In fact, it's a myth. Studies have repeatedly shown that eating extra protein produces no further gains in strength, muscle mass or size (Tipton and Wolfe, 2007). This can be achieved only through consistent and intense training in combination with a "normal" protein intake and healthy diet. Protein over and above a young athlete's requirements will be used as fuel or excreted, not converted into muscle.

Is the timing of protein intake important?

The timing of protein intake is just as important as the amount. Studies have shown that athletes recover faster and gain more muscle when they eat some of their protein before and also straight after (within two hours) training (Phillips *et al.*, 2007). This may reduce muscle damage and reduce recovery time between training sessions.

Ideally, they should have a snack or meal containing both carbohydrate and protein in a ratio of four to one. This can be obtained from a 200 ml glass of semi-skimmed milk with a banana, for example (32 g carbohydrate, 8 g protein). Thereafter, divide their daily protein intake between three meals and one or two healthy snacks.

Can vegetarians do well in sport without eating meat?

Lots of people imagine that, without meat, young athletes can't get enough protein to train hard and build muscle. But there's no evidence for this whatsoever. In fact, there are plenty of highly successful vegetarian athletes. Protein isn't available only from meat. A report from the American Dietetic Association and American College of Sports Medicine published in 2000 stated that meat and fish are not essential for athletic performance. Many scientific studies have shown that a vegetarian diet can meet the needs of competitive athletes (e.g. Craig *et al.*, 2009). The American College of Sports Medicine advises that vegetarian athletes should eat around 10 percent more protein than non-vegetarians because plant proteins are less well digested than animal proteins (Rodriquez *et al.*, 2009).

If an athlete omits meat then they would need to substitute other kinds of protein: milk, yogurt, cheese, eggs, beans, lentils, nuts, seeds and cereals. The key is to include a variety of different protein foods throughout the day in order to get a better overall balance of amino acids (the building blocks of proteins). This is called "protein complementation." For example, combining grains and legumes (such as rice and beans) gives a higher intake of all the amino acids needed to make new body proteins than eating, say, grains or legumes on their own. Try to include foods from at least two of the following four groups:

1 Legumes: beans, lentils, peas.
2 Grains: bread, pasta, rice, oats, breakfast cereals, corn, rye.
3 Nuts and seeds: peanuts, cashews, almonds, sunflower seeds, sesame seeds, pumpkin seeds.
4 Dairy products: milk, cheese, yogurt, eggs.

VEGGIE OPTIONS

Going vegetarian doesn't mean replacing meat with vegetables. It may mean a little extra planning, trying new foods and spending a little more time preparing meals. Here are some suggested vegetarian meals combining two or more protein foods:

- Baked beans on toast
- Pasta with cheese
- Bean chili with rice
- Peanut butter sandwich
- Lentil soup with a roll
- Dahl (lentils) with naan bread
- Stir-fried tofu and vegetable dish with rice
- Wholegrain cereal with milk

The North American Vegetarian Society's website (www.navs-online.org) has a section for young vegetarians with useful information about meat-free diets, as well as lots of easy recipes you can make.

Could protein supplements benefit young athletes?

Protein supplements, such as protein shakes and bars, are unnecessary for young athletes. Although athletic children need more protein than average children, they should still be able to obtain their protein from food rather than supplements. Even the most active would need no more than 80–90 g protein a day, an amount that can easily be provided by a balanced diet containing enough energy (calories) to meet the athlete's training needs, as well as two or three servings of meat, fish, dairy and poultry. Consumption of protein supplements to get a protein intake beyond this level does not make sense economically or scientifically (Tarnopolsky, 2007).

How important is fat for young athletes?

Fat is important for everyone's health, including athletes. It's used to provide energy for day-to-day activities as well as for sports and exercise. Fat in food not only provides an energy source (9 kcal per gram), but also provides the essential fatty acids (*see* below) and the fat-soluble vitamins A, D and E.

A certain amount of body fat is **vital** for the body to function normally and healthily. It is used for making body cell membranes, brain tissue, nerve sheaths, bone marrow and protective layers that cushion the organs.

How much body fat should young athletes have?

There is no ideal level of body fat an athlete should aim for but, generally, a low body fat percentage means better sports performance. A high body fat level will reduce speed and efficiency of movement. But that's not to say that athletes should try to get as lean as possible – too little body fat can be dangerous for their health and even result in a drop in performance. For female athletes, low body fat levels cause a drop in estrogen levels, a loss of bone mass and increased risk of fracture. For each person there is an optimal fat percentage at which they will perform at their best (*see* Chapter 3, page 65).

How much fat should young athletes eat?

In the UK, the amount of fat recommended for health for the general population is 15–35 percent of energy, or a maximum of 70 g a day for people consuming 2000 kcal, 95 g a day for people consuming 2500 kcal. Higher intakes may increase the risk of developing obesity, high blood cholesterol levels, heart disease and stroke.

But for athletes there is no specific guidance. The International Olympic Committee (IOC) and International Association of Athletic Federations (IAAF) both recommend that athletes focus their efforts on getting enough carbohydrate and protein (IOC, 2003; IAAF, 2007). The balance of their calorie intake should come from fats – ideally "good" rather than "bad" fats (*see* "What are good and bad fats?", below). These will provide numerous health benefits as well as an energy source. You should not be overly concerned about a young athlete's fat intake. Remember that they have higher energy needs – and therefore fat requirements – than most people, as they are growing and developing as well as training.

THE FAT CONTENT OF VARIOUS FOODS

Food	Fat content
Plain hamburger (110 g)	10 g
French fries (average portion, 110 g)	17 g
2 chocolate digestive cookies	8 g
1 chocolate bar	12 g
1 packet (30 g) of potato chips	10 g
1 chocolate-coated granola bar (24 g)	7 g
2 hotdogs (2 x 20 g)	8 g
1 small cupcake or muffin (30 g)	4 g

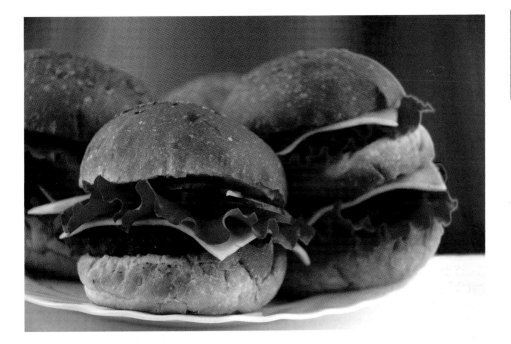

What are "good" and "bad" fats?

"Good" fats are the unsaturated fats – the monounsaturates and polyunsaturates, found in nuts, seeds, olives (and their oils) and fish.

"Bad" fats are saturated fats and trans fats, which have been linked to increased risk of heart disease and cancer.

Table 1.11 Good and bad fats

Good fats	Bad fats
Monounsaturated fats: olive oil, rapeseed oil, avocados, nuts, peanut butter	*Saturated fats:* fatty meats, burgers, hot dogs, butter, palm oil, cookies, cakes, cheese
Polyunsaturated fats: sunflower oil, corn oil, sunflower margarine, nuts, seeds	*Trans fats:* some margarines and spreads, cookies, pastries, pies, cakes, fast food, fried food
Omega-3 fats: sardines, salmon, walnuts, pumpkin seeds, omega-3 eggs	

Good fats

Monounsaturated fats help lower "bad" LDL (low-density lipoprotein) cholesterol levels while maintaining levels of "good" HDL (high-density lipoprotein), which helps cut heart disease and cancer risk. They are found in olive oil, rapeseed and soya oil, avocados, nuts, peanut butter and seeds.

Polyunsaturated fats include omega-3 and omega-6 fats.

Omega-3 fatty acids include alpha linolenic acid (ALA, found in walnuts, pumpkin seeds, flaxseeds and rapeseed oil), eicosapentanoic acid (EPA) and docosahexanoic acid (DHA), the latter two are both found only in oily fish (sardines, mackerel, salmon, fresh tuna, trout, herring). In the body, ALA can be converted into EPA and DHA, which are needed for the proper functioning of the brain, protect against heart disease and stroke, and may help prevent memory loss and treat depression. For athletes, they help increase the delivery of oxygen to muscles, improve endurance, speed recovery, and reduce inflammation and joint stiffness. The minimum requirement is 0.9 g per day, which can come from one portion (140 g) of oily fish a week or one tablespoon of omega-3-rich oil daily.

Omega-6 fatty acids include linolenic acid and gamma linolenic acid (GLA) found in sunflower, safflower, corn, groundnut and olive oils, and margarine-type spreads made with them, peanuts and peanut butter, and sunflower and sesame seeds. Most children get plenty of omega-6s but not enough omega-3s.

Bad fats

Saturated fats are found in animal fats as well as products made with palm oil. They have no beneficial role in the body (apart from being a source of energy). They raise blood cholesterol levels and increase the risk of heart disease. However, it would be impractical to cut them out altogether, so young athletes should try to stick to an intake less than the GDA: 30 g for males and 20 g for females.

Main sources include fatty meats, full-fat dairy products, butter, lard, palm oil and palm kernel oil (both labelled as "vegetable fat" on foods), and cookies, cakes and desserts made with palm or palm kernel oil or "vegetable fat".

Trans fats are formed artificially during the commercial process of hydrogenation, which converts unsaturated oils into solid spreads (hydrogenated fats or oils) for making cookies, desserts and pastry. Trans fats increase LDL ("bad") cholesterol levels and lower HDL ("good") cholesterol, and harden and stiffen the arteries, which increases the risk of heart disease.

Young athletes should try to avoid these fats completely by checking for hydrogenated oils and partially hydrogenated oils on the ingredients list on food packages.

What do vitamins and minerals do?

Vitamins and minerals are substances that are needed in tiny amounts to enable the body to work properly and prevent illness. There are 13 different vitamins, which are involved in numerous processes, including energy production, nerve and muscle function, the immune system, brain function, and healthy growth and development. Some vitamins – the B vitamins and vitamin C – must be provided by the diet each day, as they cannot be stored. The 15 minerals have mainly structural roles, such as bone strength, and regulatory roles, such as fluid balance and muscle contraction. Table 1.12 gives more details of the functions, requirements, sources and side-effects of vitamins and minerals.

WHAT ARE RDAs?

You'll see recommended daily amounts (RDAs) on food and supplement labels, which are estimates of nutrient requirements set by the USDA and designed to cover the needs of the majority (97 percent) of the general population. The amounts are designed to prevent deficiency symptoms, but also allow for storage and individual variation, as well as covering differences in needs from one person to the next. They do not necessarily cover the needs of people who are physically very active, so regard them as a rough guide only.

Do athletes need extra vitamins and minerals?

Athletes' requirements for most vitamins and minerals are higher than those of non-active people. Many of them are involved in producing energy and helping the body recover after exercise. Some are involved in repairing cells broken down during exercise, making new muscle tissue, making red blood cells and protecting cells against the harmful free radicals produced during exercise.

The best way for young athletes to get their vitamins and minerals is by eating a nutrient-rich diet, rather than taking supplements. Make sure they include lots of fruit and vegetables – at least five daily portions – and wholegrain cereals (rather than white versions), and keep low-nutrient foods such as sugary snacks, fried foods, fast foods and soft drinks to a minimum.

Can vitamin and mineral supplements improve their performance?

It is tempting to believe that supplements will benefit an athlete's performance but, in fact, there's little scientific evidence to support their use (IOC, 2004; Lukaski, 2004). According to a 2009 review of evidence, supplements are not needed if athletes are eating a varied diet that matches their energy needs (Rodriquez *et al.*, 2009). Only if their diet is unbalanced (e.g. lacking fresh fruit and vegetables; or any major food group), should you consider supplements. In general, young athletes should aim to get their vitamins and minerals from their diet rather than from supplements. Nutrients are absorbed better from food, where there are also other important components such as fiber, protein and essential fats. Supplements are not a substitute for an unhealthy diet.

Table 1.12 A guide to vitamins and minerals

Vitamin/ mineral	How much?*	Why is it needed?	What happens if we get too little?	What are the best food sources?	Side-effects of excessive intake?
Vitamin A	700 mcg (boys) 600 mcg (girls) FSA recommends 1500 mcg max.	Needed for growth and development in children; helps vision in dim light; keeps the skin, hair and eyes healthy; keeps the linings of organs such as the lungs and digestive tract healthy; helps the body to fight infections	Poor vision, dry skin, impaired growth in children, and an increased susceptibility to infection	Liver, cheese, oily fish, eggs, butter, margarine	Liver and bone damage; can harm unborn children in pregnant women (avoid during pregnancy)
Beta-carotene	No official RNI SUL = 7 mg	Converts into vitamin A, a powerful antioxidant that may protect against certain cancers and heart disease		Dark-green vegetables such as spinach and watercress, and yellow, orange and red fruits such as carrots, tomatoes, dried apricots, sweet potatoes and mangoes	Excessive doses of beta-carotene can cause harmless orange tinge to skin; reversible

Vitamin/ mineral	How much?*	Why is it needed?	What happens if we get too little?	What are the best food sources?	Side-effects of excessive intake?
Thiamin	0.9 mg (11–14 y/o boys) 1.1 mg (15–18 y/o boys) 0.7 mg (11–14 y/o girls) 0.8 mg (15–18 y/o girls) no SUL; FSA recommends 100 mg	Converts carbohydrates to energy; keeps nervous system and the heart healthy	Tiredness, poor appetite, headaches, muscle fatigue, poor concentration, depression, irritability and heart problems	Wholegrain bread, fortified breakfast cereals, nuts, legumes, meat	Excess is excreted, so toxicity is rare
Riboflavin	0.9 mg (11–14 y/o boys) 1.1 mg (15–18 y/o boys) 0.7 mg (11–14 y/o girls) 0.8 mg (15–18 y/o girls) no SUL; FSA recommends 40 mg	Converts carbohydrates, fats and protein into energy	Poor wound healing, and skin, eye and mouth problems such as watery, bloodshot eyes, flaky and dry skin, chapped lips and a sore tongue	Milk and dairy products, meat, eggs	Excess is excreted (producing yellow urine), so toxicity is rare

Vitamin/ mineral	How much?*	Why is it needed?	What happens if we get too little?	What are the best food sources?	Side-effects of excessive intake?
Niacin	15 mg (11–14 y/o boys) 18 mg (15–18 y/o boys) 12 mg (11–14 y/o girls) 14 mg (15–18 y/o girls) SUL = 17 mg	Converts carbohydrates, fats and protein into energy	Skin problems, weakness, fatigue and loss of appetite	Meat and organ meats, nuts, milk and dairy products, eggs, wholegrain cereals	Excess is excreted; high doses may cause hot flushes
Folate	200 mcg for 11–18 y/o boys and girls	Formation of red blood cells; works with vitamin B12 for growth and the reproduction of cells	Tiredness, apathy and depression	Dark-green leafy vegetables, oranges, fortified breakfast cereals and bread, yeast extract, nuts and legumes	May mask symptoms of a B12 deficiency

Vitamin/ mineral	How much?*	Why is it needed?	What happens if we get too little?	What are the best food sources?	Side-effects of excessive intake?
Vitamin C	35 mg for 11–14 y/o boys and girls 40 mg for 15–18 y/o boys and girls SUL = 1000 mg	Formation of collagen, which constitutes connective tissue; needed for healthy bones, teeth, blood vessels, gums and teeth; promotes immune function; helps iron absorption	Loss of appetite, muscle cramps, dry skin, bleeding gums, bruising, nose bleeds, infections and poor wound healing; in severe cases scurvy develops	Fruit and vegetables (e.g. raspberries, blackcurrants, kiwi fruit, oranges, peppers, broccoli, cabbage, tomatoes)	Excess is excreted; doses over 2 g may lead to diarrhea and excess urine formation; high doses (> 2 g) may cause vitamin C to behave as a pro-oxidant (enhance free radical damage)
Vitamin D	No RNI SUL = 25 mcg	Needed for strong bones (with calcium and phosphorus), helps to absorb calcium, and may help to prevent osteoporosis in later life	Reduced absorption of calcium (increasing the risk of osteoporosis); deficiency in babies and toddlers leads to soft bones and the development of rickets	Sunlight, oily fish, eggs, liver, fortified breakfast cereals and margarine	Toxicity rare; very high doses may cause high blood pressure, irregular heart beat; excessive thirst

Vitamin/ mineral	How much?*	Why is it needed?	What happens if we get too little?	What are the best food sources?	Side-effects of excessive intake?
Vitamin E	15 mg (14–18 y/o boys) 15 mg (14–18 y/o girls)	Antioxidant that helps protect against heart disease; promotes normal cell growth and development	Deficiency is rare	Vegetable oils, margarine, oily fish, nuts, seeds, egg yolk, avocado	Toxicity is rare
Calcium	1000 mg (11–18 y/o boys) 800 mg (11–18 y/o girls) SUL = 1500 mg	Builds bone and teeth; blood clotting; nerve and muscle function	Increased risk of osteoporosis	Milk and dairy products, sardines, dark-green leafy vegetables, legumes, nuts and seeds	High intakes may interfere with absorption of other minerals; take with magnesium and vitamin D
Iron	11.3 mg (11–18 y/o boys) 14.8 mg (11–18 y/o girls) SUL = 17 mg	Formation of red blood cells; oxygen transport; prevents anemia	Iron deficiency; anemia	Meat and organ meats, wholegrain cereals, fortified breakfast cereals, legumes, green leafy vegetables	Constipation, stomach discomfort; avoid unnecessary supplementation – may increase free radical damage

Vitamin/ mineral	How much?*	Why is it needed?	What happens if we get too little?	What are the best food sources?	Side-effects of excessive intake?
Zinc	9.0 mg (11–14 y/o boys) 9.5 mg (15–18 y/o boys) 9.0 mg (11–14 y/o girls) 7.0 mg (15–18 y/o girls) SUL = 25 mg	Healthy immune system; wound healing; skin cell growth	Loss of taste; frequent infections; poor wound healing	Eggs, wholegrain cereals, meat, milk and dairy products	Interferes with absorption of iron and copper

Notes

1. mg = milligram (1000 mg = 1 gram)
2. mcg = microgram (1000 mcg = 1 mg)
3. SUL = safe upper limit recommended by the Expert Group on Vitamins and Minerals, an independent advisory committee to the Food Standards Agency (FSA).
* The amount needed is given as the reference nutrient intake (RNI) (Department of Health, 1991). This is the amount of a nutrient that should cover the needs of 97 percent of the population. Athletes may need more.

Should young athletes take antioxidant supplements?

Many vitamins and minerals act as antioxidant nutrients. These include beta-carotene, vitamin C and vitamin E, zinc and selenium. Along with enzymes produced in the body, and plant compounds called phytonutrients, they help prevent or reduce cell damage caused by free radicals (*see* the box entitled "What are free radicals?"). While young athletes may need more antioxidants than the general population (as the body produces more free radicals during exercise), they don't have to take supplements. That's because the body steps up its production of antioxidant enzymes in response to regular exercise. However, it's also a good idea to eat plenty of foods that contain high levels of antioxidant nutrients: fruit, vegetables, nuts and seeds. Scientists have found that supplements don't work as well as the naturally occurring antioxidants in foods.

WHAT ARE FREE RADICALS?

Free radicals are destructive elements, which are produced all the time as a normal part of cell processes. In small numbers they are not a problem but, in larger numbers, they can cause build-up in the arteries, and increase the risk of thrombosis, heart disease and cancer. They are also thought to be partly responsible for post-exercise muscle soreness. Antioxidants neutralize them and therefore an antioxidant-rich diet may help protect against these conditions and promote faster recovery after exercise.

Can antioxidant supplements improve athletic performance?

A review of studies presented at the IOC Consensus Conference on sports nutrition concluded that there is limited evidence that antioxidant supplements improve performance (IOC, 2003).

Instead, encourage young athletes to eat five portions of fruit and vegetables each day, including a range of different colors – the more intense the color, the higher the antioxidant content – as well as foods such as avocados, nuts, oily fish and pure vegetable oils for their vitamin E content.

Salt and athletic performance

WHY DO YOUNG ATHLETES NEED SALT?

The body needs a small amount of salt for normal body functions. It helps to control the movement of fluid between cells, the amount of blood circulating, the absorption and transport of nutrients, and the action of muscles. Athletes lose some salt each day in sweat and urine, which is easily replaced by the food they eat. We actually need only 1.4 g a day, considerably lower than the average daily intake of 8.6 g and the daily limit recommended by the USDA (2.3 g).

Do young athletes need extra salt?

Although athletes lose some salt (sodium) in sweat during exercise, this is a relatively small amount, on average around 1.2 g salt (0.5 g sodium) per 1 liter of sweat, equivalent to one to two hours' hard training. Clearly, the amount of sweat produced depends on the temperature and humidity, as well as the duration and intensity of exercise.

For most young athletes, there's no need to add extra salt to their diet. Salt losses in sweat are easily replaced by a normal diet. Practically all foods contain some salt naturally (even fruit and vegetables). Eating too much rather than too little is more likely to be the problem.

How much salt should young athletes consume?

Most people eat too much salt from foods, such as bread, sauces, ready-made soup, ham, bacon, frozen meals, cheese, breakfast cereals and chips. The dietary guidelines recommend no more than 2.3 g a day for children and teenagers. This is because too much salt can raise blood pressure, which increases the risk of stroke, heart and kidney disease. Although high blood pressure is more common in older adults, it can also develop in children. As well as cutting down on salty foods everyone should also eat plenty of fruit, vegetables and low-fat dairy products for potassium, magnesium and calcium – three minerals that help to counter the effects of too much salt.

Why do commercial sports drinks contain sodium?

Makers of sports drinks claim that the sodium in the drinks replaces the losses in sweat. However, young athletes can get plenty of sodium from food eaten after exercise. The reason manufacturers add sodium to sports drinks is to stimulate thirst and encourage drinking. Sodium also has an anti-diuretic effect, reducing urine production and helping the body retain more fluid. This may be useful for promoting recovery after exercise (*see* Chapter 2, page 55).

WATCH OUT FOR HIDDEN SALT

Three-quarters (75 percent) of the salt we eat comes from processed food, so you might not realize how much salt young athletes are eating.

Food	Salt content
Bran flakes (small portion, 30 g)	0.5 g
Beef hotdogs (two average)	2.3 g
Bacon (2 x 27 g slices)	2.0 g
Ham (2 x 23 g slices)	1.4 g
Tomato soup (½ tin)	1.0 g
Pasta sauce (½ jar, 170 g)	1.8 g
Pizza (one restaurant pizza, 300 g)	3.0–4.0 g
Chips (one packet, 35 g)	0.5 g
Cheese (one slice, 25 g)	0.4 g

How to plan a healthy diet for young athletes

When it comes to planning meals and snacks, it's easier to think in terms of food groups than nutrients. The idea is that each group of foods provides a similar range of nutrients – dairy products, for example, contain high levels of calcium and protein. By eating the recommended number of portions of each food group each day, the young athlete should meet his or her requirements for key nutrients. For best health, try to include a wide variety of foods from each food group. That way, they stand a better chance of getting more nutrients.

I have devised a "fitness food pyramid," which is based on the USDA's MyPlate, to help athletes plan their diet. The main difference between the fitness food pyramid and MyPlate is that the former includes six instead of five food groups – the healthy fats group is extra. While MyPlate is designed for the general population aged two years and over, the fitness food pyramid is designed for athletes who have higher energy needs, and so recommends more generous portion sizes and a higher number of daily portions from certain food groups.

The fitness food pyramid

The components of the fitness food pyramid are described below (*see* also Table 1.13).

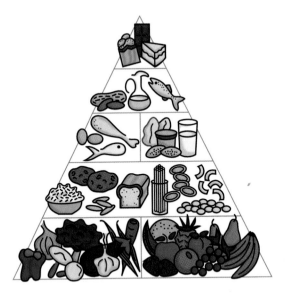

Fruit and vegetables
At least 5 portions a day

Fruit and vegetables contain vitamins, minerals, fiber, antioxidants and phyto-nutrients, which are vital for health, immunity and peak performance.

Grains and starches
4–6+ portions a day

The foods in this group – bread, breakfast cereals, rice, pasta, oatmeal and potatoes – provide high levels of carbohydrate. More active people will need to eat more portions or bigger portions to meet their energy needs. Aim for mostly wholegrain versions of cereals, i.e. wholegrain bread, breakfast cereals and pasta instead of "white" versions, as these have a higher content of fiber, iron and B vitamins. The portion sizes in this group are about twice those recommended in MyPlate.

Calcium-rich foods
2–4 portions a day

The foods in this group include dairy products, nuts, legumes and canned fish; they provide high amounts of calcium, which is needed for strong bones.

Protein-rich foods
2–4 portions a day

This group includes lean meat, chicken, turkey, fish, eggs, beans, lentils, dairy products, soya and meat-substitutes such as Quorn; these provide protein as well as various different vitamins and minerals.

Healthy fats
1–2 portions a day

Omega-3 and omega-6 unsaturated fats found in nuts, seeds, rapeseed oil, olive oil, flaxseed oil, sunflower oil and oily fish are important for heart health, and for good performance and recovery after exercise.

Foods and drinks high in fats and/or sugar

These foods – cookies, cakes, puddings, sugary drinks, chocolate and chips – should be regarded as treats. As they provide energy but few nutrients other than fat or sugar, try to limit them to about three portions a day. They should not take the place of more nutrient-dense foods – make sure young athletes eat the recommended number of portions of the other food groups first.

Table 1.13 The fitness food pyramid

Food group	Number of portions each day	Food	Portion size
1a Vegetables	3–5	*1 portion = 80 g (about the amount you can hold in the palm of your hand)*	
		Broccoli, cauliflower	2–3 florets
		Carrots	1 carrot
		Other vegetables	2 tablespoons
		Tomatoes	5 cherry tomatoes
1b Fruit	2–4	*1 portion = 80 g (about the size of a tennis ball)*	
		Apple, pear, peach, banana	1 medium fruit

Food group	Number of portions each day	Food	Portion size
		Plum, kiwi fruit, satsuma	1–2 fruits
		Strawberries	8–10
		Grapes	12–16
		Canned fruit	3 tablespoons
		Fruit juice	1 medium glass
2 Grains and potatoes	4–6+	*1 portion = about the size of your clenched fist*	
		Bread	2 slices (60 g)
		Roll/bagel/wrap	1 item (60 g)
		Pasta or rice	5 tablespoons (180 g)
		Breakfast cereal	1 bowl (40–50 g)
		Potatoes, sweet potatoes, yams	1 fist-sized (150 g)
3 Calcium-rich foods	2–4	*1 portion = 200 ml milk*	
		Milk (dairy or calcium-fortified soya milk)	1 medium cup (200 ml)
		Cheese	Size of 4 dice (40 g)
		Tofu	Size of 4 dice (60 g)
		Yogurt	1 container (150 ml)
4 Protein-rich foods	2–4	*1 portion = size of a deck of cards (70 g)*	
		Lean meat	3 slices

Food group	Number of portions each day	Food	Portion size
		Poultry	2 medium slices/ 1 chicken or turkey breast
		Fish	1 filet (115–140 g)
		Eggs	2
		Lentils/beans	5 tablespoons (150 g)
		Tofu/soya burger or sausage	1–2
5 Healthy fats and oils	1–2	*1 portion = 1 tablespoon* Nuts and seeds	2 tablespoons (25 g)
		Seed oils, nut oils	1 tablespoon (15 ml)
		Avocado	Half avocado
		Oily fish*	Deck of cards (140 g)
6 Foods and drinks high in sugars and/or fats	< 3	Cookies	2
		Chips	1 bag
		Chocolate	30 g (6 squares)
		Granola bar	1 bar
		Cake	1 cupcake
		Sugary drink	500 ml

* Oily fish is very rich in essential fats so just 1 portion a week would cover a young athlete's needs

References

Boisseau, N. *et al.*, "Protein Requirements in Male Adolescent Soccer Players," *European Journal of Applied Physiology*, May, 100(1) (2007), pp. 27–33.

Burke, D.G. *et al.*, "Glycaemic Index – a New Tool in Sports Nutrition," *International Journal of Sport Nutrition*, 8 (1998), pp. 401–415.

Craig, W.J. *et al.*, "Position of the American Dietetic Association: Vegetarian Diets," *Journal of the American Dietetic Association*, 109(7) (2009), pp. 1266–1282.

Department of Health, *Dietary Reference Values for Food Energy and Nutrients for the United Kingdom* (HMSO, 1991).

International Association of Athletic Federations (IAAF), *Nutrition for Athletics: The 2007 IAAF Consensus Statement* (IAAF, 2007).

International Olympic Committee (IOC), "Consensus on Sports Nutrition, 2003," *Journal of Sports Science*, 22(1) (2003), p. x.

Lukaski, H.C., "Vitamin and Mineral Status: Effects on Physical Performance," *Nutrition*, 20 (2004), pp. 632–644.

Macdougall, J.D. *et al.*, "Maximal Aerobic Capacity of Canadian School Children: Prediction Based on Age-Related Oxygen Cost of Running," *Journal of Sports Medicine*, 4 (1982), pp. 194–198.

Phillips, S.M. *et al.*, "A Critical Examination of Dietary Protein Requirements, Benefits and Excesses in Athletes," *International Journal of Sport Nutrition and Exercise Metabolism*, 17 (2007), pp. 58–78.

Rodriquez, N.R. *et al.*, "Position of the American Dietetic Association, Dietitians of Canada, and the American College of Sports Medicine: Nutrition and Athletic Performance," *Journal of the American Dietetic Association*, 109(3) (2009), pp. 509–527.

Schofield, W.N. *et al.*, "Basal Metabolic Rate – Review and Prediction," *Human Nutrition: Clinical Nutrition*, 39(suppl.) (1985), pp. 1–96.

Scientific Advisory Committee on Nutrition, *Salt and Health* (The Stationery Office, 2003).

Tarnopolsky, M., "Building Muscle," Sport Nutrition Conference (Birmingham University, 2007).

Tipton, K. and Wolfe, R., "Protein Needs and Amino Acids for Athletes," *Journal of Sports Science*, 22(1) (2007), pp. 65–79.

Wu, C.L. and Williams, C., "A Low Glycaemic Index Meal Before Exercise Improves Endurance Running Capacity in Men," *Journal of Sports Nutrition and Exercise Metabolism*, 16 (2006), pp. 510–527.

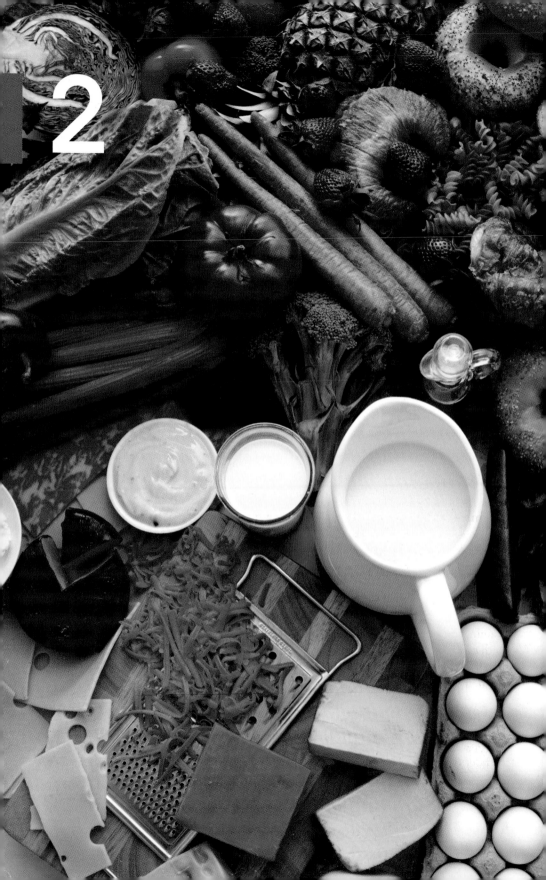

2

EATING FOR SPORT

Eating the right type of food and drinking enough fluid before, during and after each training session will help young athletes perform better, reduce fatigue and prevent them getting ill.

This chapter will explain the key nutritional strategies that can be used to improve their training sessions. These center around providing sufficient fuel for the muscles, maintaining hydration, and promoting post-exercise recovery. They can best be achieved by considering sports nutrition in three distinct phases:

1 before training;
2 during training;
3 after training.

This chapter will also provide some practical guidelines for pre-training meals, snacks and drinks; some suggestions for eating and drinking during training; and, finally, recommendations for what to eat and drink after training to promote fast recovery.

Before training

It's important that young athletes begin each training session fully fueled and properly hydrated. This will allow them to exercise harder and for longer. Many studies have shown that a carbohydrate-rich diet before exercise results in increased endurance and better performance (e.g. Rodriquez, *et al.*, 2009). Conversely, an inadequate carbohydrate intake results in low muscle stores and reduced endurance. It increases the risk of early fatigue and poor performance. The athlete may struggle to keep up the pace, they may lag behind their teammates, they may feel weak, and they may have to stop training before the end of the session. It's rather like setting off in a car on a long journey with only half a tank of gas. Without enough fuel, you won't be able to drive so far and you'll have to reduce your speed to conserve what little fuel you have. On the other hand, if you set off with plenty of fuel you'll be able to go faster and further.

WHAT IS THE PURPOSE OF THE PRE-EXERCISE MEAL?

The pre-exercise meal should provide the athlete with sustained energy, prevent them from feeling hungry during training, and be easily digested.

When should young athletes eat before training?

The optimal time for the pre-exercise meal is two to four hours before exercise (Hargreaves *et al.*, 2004). Carbohydrate in this meal will help top up muscle and liver glycogen levels and enhance performance during training or competition. If young athletes leave a longer gap than four hours, then they will almost certainly feel hungry during training, tired and light-headed. On the other hand, if they eat too much too close to training, then they may feel uncomfortable, "heavy" or nauseous, and unable to train hard as the blood supply diverts to the digestive organs instead of the muscles.

In practice, the exact timing of their pre-exercise meal will probably depend on constraints such as school hours, travel, homework and training session times. Try to plan meals as best you can around these commitments. If the training session starts at 7 o'clock, plan to eat at about 5 o'clock. But if the athlete must train earlier, then they should eat a smaller meal, which is easier to digest, and which will produce the same benefits. They should feel comfortable, neither full nor hungry.

If the young athlete has to train straight after school, during their lunch break or first thing in the morning, then they may not have time for a meal. Instead, they should have a smaller meal or healthy snack, and include a drink. The food eaten should be easily digestible – high in carbohydrate, low in fat – such as toast, a granola bar or a juice drink (*see* the box entitled "Pre-training snacks" for more ideas).

What should young athletes eat before training?

The pre-training meal should be based on a high-carbohydrate food such as bread, pasta, potatoes or rice. These foods have a low glycemic index (GI, *see* the box entitled "What is the glycemic index?"), which means they produce a gradual increase in blood sugar levels and give sustained energy. Studies have shown that athletes are able to exercise considerably longer after eating a low-GI meal compared with a high-GI meal (Chryssanthopoulos *et al.*, 2002). A low-GI meal helps maintain blood sugar levels, increase endurance and delay fatigue.

Include some protein in the pre-training meal: chicken, fish, cheese, egg, beans, lentils or nuts. This will assist in lowering the overall GI of the meal as well as help reduce muscle breakdown during exercise and improve performance (Kerksick *et al.*, 2008). Avoid too much fat as this takes longer to digest and may make the athlete feel uncomfortable during training. Fried foods, hotdogs, burgers and fries should be off the menu before training!

Oatmeal, cereal with milk, a baked potato with beans or a light pasta meal would be suitable pre-workout meals (*see* the box entitled "Pre-training meals" for more suggestions).

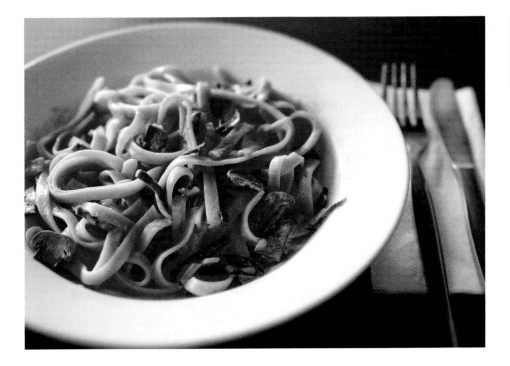

PRE-TRAINING MEALS

- Baked potato with cheese, tuna or baked beans, plus salad
- Pasta with tomato-based sauce or pesto, a little cheese and some vegetables
- Rice, pasta or noodles with chicken, fish or beans, and vegetables
- A bowl of wholegrain breakfast cereal with milk and banana
- Oatmeal with milk, honey and raisins
- Lentil/vegetable or chicken soup with wholewheat bread
- Wholewheat sandwich/roll/wrap filled with tuna/cheese/chicken/peanut butter and salad

PRE-TRAINING SNACKS

If there is not time for a meal, the young athlete should have a snack 30 minutes before training, with a drink of water.

- One or two bananas (or other fresh fruit)
- A handful of dried fruit and nuts
- One or two granola bars
- A container of fruit yogurt and some fresh fruit
- One or two slices of bread or toast with honey
- Two or three mini-pancakes
- A smoothie (home-made or ready made)
- Rice cakes with peanut butter or a little cheese

WHAT IS THE GLYCEMIC INDEX?

The glycemic index (GI) is a ranking of foods from 0 to 100 based on their immediate effect on blood sugar levels. Glucose has a GI of 100. It's a measure of how quickly the food turns into glucose in the bloodstream. Foods with a high GI (above 70) cause a rapid rise in blood sugar levels. These include many refined ("white") starchy foods – such as cornflakes, white bread and white rice – as well as sugary foods such as soft drinks, cookies and candy.

Foods with a low GI (below 55) produce a slower and smaller blood sugar rise. These include beans, lentils, wholegrain breads, muesli, fresh fruit and dairy products. Foods that contain no carbohydrate – meat, fish, chicken, eggs, oil, butter and margarine – have no GI value.

Table 2.1 lists examples of low-, medium- and high-GI foods.

Table 2.1 Low-, medium- and high-GI foods

Low-GI foods	Medium-GI foods	High-GI foods
Pasta	Brown and basmati rice	White bread and rolls, French bread and bagels
Beans and lentils	Pizza	Most breakfast cereals, e.g. cornflakes, Rice Krispies, Cocoa Puffs
Milk and yogurt	Flatbread	White rice

Low-GI foods	Medium-GI foods	High-GI foods
Peas	Pita bread	Most wholewheat bread
Most vegetables, e.g. cucumber, broccoli	Boiled potatoes	Mashed and baked potatoes
		Doughnuts
Most fresh fruit, e.g. apples, pears, bananas, grapes, kiwi fruit	Canned fruit	French fries
Dried apricots	Ice cream	Jam and sugar
Nuts	Raisins	Soft drinks
Oatmeal, bran cereals and muesli	Granola bars	Candy
Multigrain bread	Digestive cookies	Most cookies

Can sugar provide a pre-exercise energy boost?

I see lots of young athletes consuming sugary foods and drinks just before training, in the belief that the sugar in these products will help them train harder and longer. Although sugar is a fuel, eating too much of it can cause rapid fluctuations in blood sugar levels and, ironically, make athletes feel more tired. Sugar-rich foods and drinks produce a rapid rise in blood sugar levels, which in turn triggers the release of insulin to remove sugar from the bloodstream. Lots of sugar makes the body produce lots of insulin, which can result in low blood sugar levels, light-headedness, nausea and early fatigue during exercise. Rather than giving them extra energy, sugar may sap their energy!

They should avoid this by consuming only small amounts of sugar before exercise – less than 25 g generally produces a moderate increase in blood sugar – or opting for a food or drink with a lower GI. If they need a pre-training energy boost, it's safer to choose foods such as bananas, dried fruit and granola bars that won't play havoc with blood sugar levels.

IF YOUNG ATHLETES HAVE TO TRAIN FIRST THING IN THE MORNING BUT DON'T FEEL HUNGRY, SHOULD THEY FORCE THEMSELVES TO EAT?

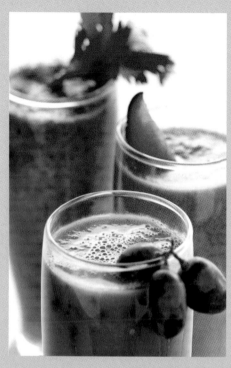

This is a bit of a dilemma because it is hard to make yourself eat when you aren't hungry, yet eating something will give the young athlete more energy for training, increase their endurance and help them perform better! However, it is possible to overcome an early-morning lack of appetite. First, they should avoid eating a big meal the night before as this takes a long time to digest fully. Second, see if they can manage just a few bites of food and a drink of water. They probably won't have time for a big breakfast, but a small healthy snack will make a big difference to their performance. They could try a granola bar, a slice of toast, a small bowl of cereal, a couple of mini-pancakes or a banana. They should always have a drink – water is the best choice. They will have lost a lot of fluid in the night and will need to rehydrate before training.

If they really cannot face food first thing, they should have a nutritious drink, such as fruit juice, a smoothie, a milk-based drink (such as a milkshake or hot chocolate) or yogurt drink. This will provide energy to fuel their muscles during training.

Get them to persevere – they will soon get used to the feeling of food and drink in their stomach early in the morning. And they will find that they'll be able to train harder and for longer.

What should young athletes drink before training?

It's important that young athletes are fully hydrated before they start training. They will have a better chance of putting in a good performance. If they are not properly hydrated before exercise, then they risk becoming more dehydrated during the training session and suffering early fatigue. Exercise will feel much harder than usual, they will tire quicker, and they risk dehydration symptoms, such as headaches, nausea and dizziness.

Prevention is better than cure. If they train in the evening, make sure they drink plenty of water during the day. If they train early in the morning, they should have a drink as soon as they get up. They will know if they are properly hydrated from the color of their urine. It should be pale straw-colored, not deep yellow, and should not have a strong odor. Try to get them into the habit of self-monitoring their hydration status. The "pee chart" presented in Figure 2.1 provides a guide to hydration levels.

Encourage young athletes to make up for any previously incurred fluid deficits by consuming 400–600 ml about two hours before training or competition, and to continue drinking a little and often during the warm-up.

When it comes to choosing what to drink, water is one of the best ways of hydrating the body. It is rapidly absorbed – and free too. Should they opt for a sports drink? Perhaps if they haven't eaten anything – in which case the sugars in the drink will help maintain blood sugar levels and fuel the muscles. Otherwise, water is a perfectly good pre-exercise choice, together with a pre-exercise meal or snack.

How much should young athletes drink each day?

There are no official guidelines for fluid intake, although many health professionals advise drinking eight 8-ounce glasses (2 liters) per day as a general guide.

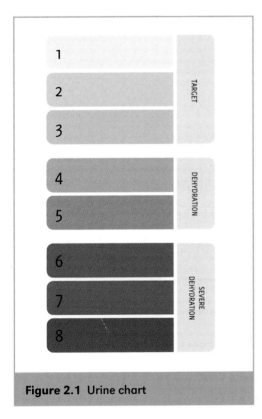

Figure 2.1 Urine chart

These recommendations don't take account of exercise, however. Young athletes will lose extra fluid through sweating during training, more in hot and humid conditions, and will certainly need to drink more than non-active people. They should drink little and often throughout the day rather than lots of water in one go. They must not ignore thirst, no matter how busy they are. The best way to tell whether they are drinking enough is from the color of their urine (Figure 2.1). If it is yellow and has a strong odor (4 or above on the pee chart), they are dehydrated and need to drink more. It should always have a color between 1 and 3 before they begin training.

Is it a good idea to have an energy drink before training?

Energy drinks have become increasingly popular among young athletes, who see them as an easy way to boost their performance. The clever marketing behind energy drinks suggests that they make you feel energetic. In fact, the opposite may be true! The term "energy" refers to the drink's high energy (or calorie) content, not its ability to boost performance. Energy drinks comprise sugar and water. The sugar content is around 10–12 g per 100 g, or 25–31 g per 250 ml can, about the same concentration as most carbonated drinks, but too concentrated for the body to absorb quickly. At such high sugar concentrations, the fluid is absorbed more slowly from energy drinks compared with water or isotonic sports drinks, which makes them an unsuitable choice for exercise. In the USA, the National Federation of State High School Associations cautions against energy drinks for hydration and warns of the potential risk of dehydration associated with them (NFHS, 2008).

Can energy drinks with caffeine enhance performance?

Many energy drinks contain caffeine (about 80 mg per 250 ml, equivalent to a cup of coffee), which is known for its ability to increase mental alertness as well as endurance performance. But don't assume that young athletes will perform better with a caffeine boost. While caffeine is considered safe for use by adults, there is little research supporting its safety and effectiveness in young athletes. High doses can also cause side-effects: an upset stomach, sleeplessness, dizziness, headaches and higher blood pressure. Everyone responds differently – young athletes may be very sensitive to caffeine so could end up feeling nauseous or suffering from "caffeine jitters" at a time when they are already nervous and anxious. Like any drug, it can also cause dependence, which means that they need more and more to get the same effect and, if they suddenly stop taking it, they may develop withdrawal symptoms (headaches, tiredness and irritability). The negative effects can outweigh potential performance benefits.

During training

During exercise the muscles produce heat, which raises the body's core temperature. To avoid the core temperature increasing excessively, the body uses a system known as thermoregulation. Heat is transferred from the muscles to the blood and blood flow to the skin is increased so that heat can escape into the atmosphere. The production of sweat and its evaporation from the skin also helps keep the body core temperature stable.

The amount of fluid lost in sweat depends on the surrounding temperature and humidity, and the intensity and duration of exercise. The warmer and more humid the conditions, and the longer and harder they exercise, the more fluid young athletes lose. Replacing these fluid losses is particularly important to prevent dehydration and its associated dangers.

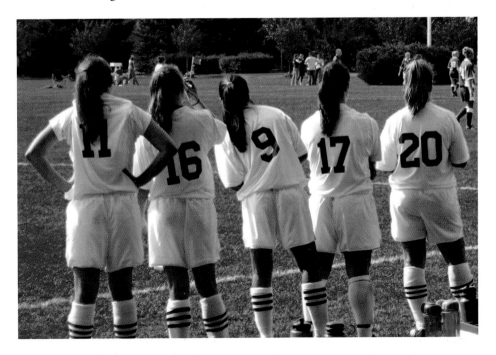

What are the signs of dehydration?

Thermoregulation is less efficient in young athletes compared with adults; they produce sweat less readily than adults and have a greater surface area to body weight ratio, so are more susceptible to dehydration.

Common symptoms of dehydration include lack of energy, nausea, early fatigue, headaches and inability to concentrate. More severe symptoms include dizziness, vomiting, disorientation and increasing weakness. Eventually this can lead to exhaustion, heat stroke and, in some cases, can be fatal. Even mild dehydration – a

2 percent loss in body weight – can impair performance, reduce stamina and strength, and increase fatigue.

WARNING SIGNS OF DEHYDRATION

Early symptoms

- Unusually lacking in energy
- Fatiguing early during exercise
- Headache
- Feeling very hot
- Skin appears flushed, and feels cool and clammy
- Passing only small volumes of dark-colored urine
- Nausea

Action: Stop exercising. Drink 100–200 ml water or sports drink every 10–15 minutes.

Advanced symptoms

- Severe headache
- Becomes dizzy or light-headed
- Appears disorientated
- Short of breath

Action: Stop exercising. Drink 100–200 ml sports drink every 10–15 minutes. Seek professional help.

What's the best way of preventing dehydration?

Prevention is certainly better than cure. Encourage young athletes to start drinking early during their training session – within the first 30 minutes – and to continue drinking at regular intervals. It takes 15–30 minutes for fluid to be absorbed into the bloodstream so athletes should not wait until they feel thirsty or experience symptoms of dehydration before they start drinking. For most people, thirst is not a reliable guide to fluid losses. They may be dehydrated by the time they feel thirsty.

Help young athletes plan their drinking strategy for each training session and competition. As a rule of thumb, they should aim to drink around 500 ml per hour – more in hot, humid weather or when exercising very strenuously. If they exercise for a shorter time or at a lower intensity, they can drink proportionally less as the risk of dehydration will be smaller. Encourage them to drink little and often during training, ideally every 15–20 minutes or whenever there is an appropriate break. Make sure they have a water bottle (or two for longer sessions) and keep it within easy reach throughout training.

To get a more accurate idea of their fluid losses, young athletes can weigh them-selves before and after training. The American College of Sports Medicine recommends that athletes should lose no more than 2 percent of their body weight during exercise (ACSM, 2007). This equates to 1.2 kg for a 60 kg person. Each 1 kg of weight loss is equivalent to 1 liter of fluid. They should try to drink at least half of this amount during training, the rest afterwards.

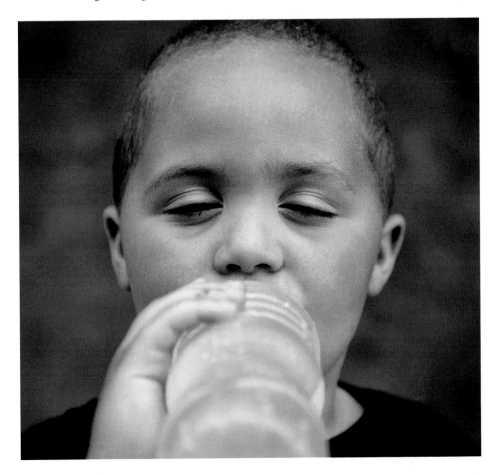

What should young athletes drink during training?

Water is fine to hydrate with during activities lasting less than an hour. The objective is to replace fluid and prevent dehydration; no extra fuel should be necessary.

However, for training sessions lasting longer than an hour, or perhaps for very intense sessions lasting 30–60 minutes, a drink that provides carbohydrate (such as diluted fruit juice or sports drink) is a better option than plain water. The advantages include:

- this provides carbohydrate to fuel the muscles during exercise (Jeukendrup, 2004);

- the carbohydrate in the drink (provided it contains between 4–8 g/100 ml) helps the fluid in the drink get absorbed more quickly (Gisolfi *et al.*, 1995);
- athletes freely drink more fluids when the drink is flavored and sweetened (Passe *et al.* 2004).

Conversely, drinking plain water doesn't refuel the muscles, it tends to satisfy thirst before athlete's fluid needs have been met, and it can lead to increased urine output (Maughan *et al.*, 1996).

How much carbohydrate should young athletes consume during training?

For exercise lasting less than an hour, it is not necessary to refuel with carbohydrates during training. The muscles should contain sufficient carbohydrate (glycogen) to fuel an hour's exercise.

When exercising for longer than an hour, refueling with carbohydrates can increase endurance and improve performance. Studies have shown that consuming between 30 and 60 g of sugar/carbohydrate per hour will help delay fatigue (IOC, 2003). This can be achieved by drinking between 500 ml and 1 liter of a drink containing 6 g sugar per 100 ml. Examples include fruit juice diluted half and half with water, or a commercial isotonic sports drink.

Sometimes athletes may prefer to eat solid food during training instead of or as well as a drink. It may be possible to eat during a training break. What they eat will probably depend on practical considerations but they should opt for high-GI carbohydrates, which convert into blood sugar rapidly, such as granola bars, bananas, dried fruit, fruit or banana bread. Make sure they also drink water to replace their fluid losses.

FOODS AND DRINKS SUITABLE FOR CONSUMPTION DURING EXERCISE LONGER THAN AN HOUR

Each of the following portions supplies 30 g carbohydrate:

- 500 ml isotonic sports drink (6 g/100 ml)
- 250 ml fruit juice mixed with 250 ml water
- 1½ granola bars (45 g)
- A handful (40 g) of raisins
- 1–2 bananas (200 g)
- 2 slices (50 g) banana bread/fruit muffin

Can commercial sports drinks help young athletes perform better?

There is a lot of marketing hype surrounding commercial sports drinks. First, it is important to understand that they are not necessary for exercise lasting less than an hour – water will provide perfectly adequate hydration. Second, even for longer sessions young athletes may get the same performance benefits by consuming other types of drinks.

So what's unique about sports drinks? They are essentially soft drinks containing one or more types of sugar (such as glucose, sucrose and maltodextrin) at a concentration between 6 and 8 g sugar/100 ml (60–80 g/liter), together with electrolytes (sodium, potassium and chloride). The sugar concentration is a little lower than that of other soft drinks, which typically contain 9–12 g per 100 ml (90–120 g/liter). At this relatively lower concentration, the sugars help the body absorb water faster than plain water. At higher concentrations, the sugars actually slow down water absorption into the body, which is why standard soft drinks would be unsuitable for rehydration during exercise. The electrolyte, sodium, in sports drinks stimulates thirst and also helps the body retain the fluid consumed.

Many studies have shown that consuming sports drinks instead of water during exercise lasting more than an hour can help improve performance (Coyle, 2004). This is due mainly to their sugar content, which helps maintain blood sugar levels and fuel the muscles. However, the major drawback of commercial sports drinks is their cost. For young athletes training daily and therefore requiring 500 ml–1 liter per session, the high price of these drinks is difficult to justify.

For a less expensive sports drink, mix fruit juice 50/50 with water or dissolve 40–60 g sugar in 1 liter of water. You may add a pinch of salt (0.5–1 g per 1 liter), although this is not essential for most types of training. These "home-made" versions of sports drinks will help athletes exercise for longer and improve performance during exercise longer than an hour.

HOW TO MAKE YOUR OWN SPORTS DRINK

- 500 ml fruit juice mixed with 500 ml water and 0.5–1 g (one-eighth of a teaspoon) salt (optional)
- 200 ml fruit juice concentrate mixed with 800 ml water and 0.5–1 g (one-eighth of a teaspoon) salt (optional)
- 40–80 g sugar and 0.5–1 g (one-eighth of a teaspoon) salt dissolved in 1 liter of warm water; add a little fruit juice for flavor, if preferred

WHAT TO DRINK DURING TRAINING

For exercise lasting less than an hour
Water

For exercise lasting more than an hour
Fruit juice diluted with an equal amount of water
Squash diluted one part to four with water
Sugar dissolved in water (40–80 g per 1 liter)
Commercial sports drink

After training

It is after, not during, exercise when the body gets stronger and fitter. There are three aspects to recovery:

1 rehydration;
2 replenishment of muscle glycogen;
3 manufacture of new muscle protein.

What is the best way to rehydrate after training?

It takes, on average, between 30 and 60 minutes for the body to rehydrate after exercise. The IOC and IAAF recommend drinking 1.2–1.5 times the weight of fluid lost during exercise (IOC, 2004; IAAF, 2007). This is to compensate for the increased urine production that accompanies drinking large volumes of fluid. If athletes weigh themselves before and after training, they can work out how much fluid they have lost. For each 1 kg of weight loss, they need to drink 1.2–1.5 liters. This should be drunk in divided amounts over an hour or so, not all in one go. Drinking a large volume is not the best way to rehydrate as it promotes diuresis (urination). The rapid expansion in blood volume and drop in blood concentration of sodium makes the body excrete more water.

Consuming a little sodium (salt) in food or drink will promote recovery because it helps the body retain the fluid drunk (Maughan and Leiper, 1995). It also stimulates thirst, encouraging athletes to drink. Young athletes can get this either from normal foods – most contain some sodium – or from sports drinks. For most cases, there's no need to consume extra salt or salty foods. But, for athletes showing signs of dehydration, they should be given a sports drink. If symptoms are quite severe (*see* page 50) they should seek medical advice and may then be offered oral or intravenous rehydration treatment.

SHOULD YOUNG ATHLETES HAVE EXTRA SALT AFTER EXERCISE TO REPLACE THEIR SWEAT LOSSES?

Some salt (sodium) is lost in sweat during exercise but this is generally quite a small amount, which can easily be replaced in a normal snack or meal, or a sports drink. Many foods contain sodium so there's no need to add extra salt. Only if young athletes have lost higher-than-normal amounts of sweat – for example, in hot, humid weather – might they benefit from a little extra salt. This can be obtained from salty foods (such as chips), which should be consumed with plenty of water, or sports drinks.

How soon should young athletes eat after training?

The sooner young athletes consume carbohydrate after training, the quicker their muscles can begin to replenish fuel stores. There is a crucial two-hour period after exercising when carbohydrate can be converted to glycogen one and a half times faster than normal (Ivy *et al.*, 1988). After this time, glycogen storage slows and returns to the normal rate.

Rapid recovery is particularly important for those athletes who train or compete twice a day. These young athletes should make sure they have a carbohydrate-rich drink or snack (*see* below) as soon as possible, ideally within 30 minutes but no later than two hours after training.

This is sometimes a problem with young athletes who train in the evening. If they arrive home late, they may not have much time to eat before bedtime or they may not feel very hungry at this time of day. In this situation, plan ahead and make sure they take refueling snacks and drinks with them to training, so that they can refuel immediately afterwards.

For those young athletes training less frequently, refueling within the 30-minute post-exercise window is less critical. Provided they consume adequate carbohydrate over each 24-hour period, they should achieve full glycogen replenishment.

What should young athletes eat after training?

The post-training meal should contain carbohydrate to replenish depleted glycogen stores, as well as protein to repair and rebuild the muscles. Ideally, young athletes should consume about 1 g carbohydrate per kg body weight (IAAF, 2007). For a 60 kg athlete, this equates to 60 g carbohydrate. They should also include a protein source in their post-training meal. Research suggests that consuming carbohydrate plus protein promotes faster recovery of glycogen stores and muscle tissue compared with a carbohydrate-only snack or meal (Tarnopolsky and MacLennan, 1997). This combination raises insulin levels in the bloodstream, and promotes the uptake of glucose and amino acids (the building blocks of protein) by the muscles. It also helps reduce muscle damage and muscle soreness, and promote muscle repair, according to a 2007 review of studies carried out by researchers at Maastricht University (Van

Loon, 2007). A 2007 study at Loughborough and Bath Universities showed that runners could run for longer following a four-hour recovery period during which they consumed a carbohydrate–protein drink (Betts *et al.*, 2007).

The ideal post-training meal or snack should contain about 10–20 g of protein to help ensure that the amino acid building blocks are on hand to repair muscle tissue damaged during training and to support the making of new muscle tissue proteins. The meal or snack should contain about four times as much carbohydrate as protein, according to University of Texas studies (Zawadski *et al.*, 1992).

What are the best foods to eat after training?

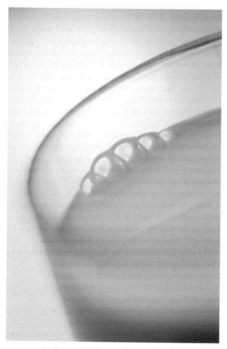

The recovery snack can be similar to the pre-training snack, perhaps with a little extra protein. Good choices include low-fat milk, flavored milk, fruit with yogurt, a granola bar with a yogurt drink, or a home-made milkshake. Flavored milk and yogurt are particularly good options because they contain carbohydrate and protein in the ideal 4:1 ratio. Milk has a naturally high electrolyte content and similar levels of carbohydrate (lactose) to those in commercial sports drinks.

Interestingly, several studies have suggested that low-fat milk may be better than sports drinks for promoting muscle recovery. A 2008 study by researchers at Northumbria University found that athletes who drank 500 ml of semi-skimmed milk or chocolate milk immediately after training had less muscle soreness and more rapid muscle recovery compared with commercial sports drinks or water (Cockburn *et al.*, 2008). Studies at Lough-borough University found that skimmed chocolate milk rehydrated athletes better than plain water or commercial sports drinks (Shireffs *et al.*, 2007). Other suitable recovery foods are shown in the box entitled "Refueling snacks and drinks."

The key is to plan ahead. Encourage young athletes to get into the habit of taking a recovery snack with them to their training session. That way, they can begin Refueling immediately. Delaying refueling by longer than 30 minutes may delay muscle recovery. For young athletes who train daily, or even twice a day, this could make a big difference to their subsequent performance. Follow the snack with a meal within two hours. This should also contain carbohydrate and protein in approximately the same 4:1 ratio, as well as healthy fats. Include fruit and vegetables in the post-training meal, aiming for a minimum of five portions throughout the day.

IS IT HEALTHY TO DRINK MILK AFTER TRAINING?

There's growing evidence which suggests that milk may be just as effective as commercial sports drinks in helping athletes recover and rehydrate. It provides fluid for rehydration, as well as protein, vitamins and minerals such as calcium, potassium and magnesium that you need to replace after strenuous exercise. Milk's high content of protein and carbohydrate can help refuel exhausted muscles. The protein in milk helps build muscle tissue, and research suggests it may reduce exercise-induced muscle damage. A 2009 study from James Madison University, USA, found that chocolate milk promoted better muscle recovery compared with a commercial sports drink (Gilson *et al.*, 2009). Football players who drank chocolate milk after training had less muscle damage and faster muscle recovery compared with those who consumed a sports drink with the same amount of calories. Flavored milk and plain milk have the advantage of additional nutrients not found in sports drinks and are therefore very good options as recovery drinks.

Refueling snacks and drinks

Each of the following provides 50–60 g carbohydrate and 10–20 g protein. They should be consumed within two hours of exercise.

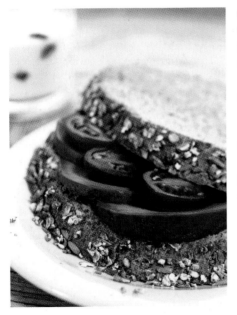

- 500 ml flavored milk
- 1 banana plus 500 ml of milk
- 2 containers (2 x 150 g) of fruit yogurt
- 1 granola bar plus 500 ml semi-skimmed milk
- A smoothie – blend 150 g yogurt, 1 banana and 150 ml fruit juice in a blender
- A cheese sandwich (2 slices of bread, 40 g cheese)
- 60 g raisins and 50 g nuts
- 4 rice cakes with 20 g peanut butter plus 200 ml orange juice

REFUELING MEALS
- Pasta with tomato sauce, grated cheese and vegetables
- Baked potato, chicken breast, broccoli and carrots
- Bean and vegetable stew with wholegrain rice
- Rice with grilled fish and steamed vegetables
- Lasagne or vegetable lasagne with salad
- Fish with vegetables
- Chili or vegetarian chili with rice and vegetables
- Dahl (lentils) with rice and vegetables
- Curry Chicken with rice and vegetables
- Mashed or baked potato with grilled salmon and salad

Menu plans

Use these menus as a basis for planning your daily menus. They have been designed to provide the optimum balance of protein, carbohydrate and fat, as well as fiber and essential vitamins and minerals, for young athletes. The menus supply approximately 2500 kcal, 3000 kcal and 3500 kcal to suit the energy needs of different individuals. There is also a plan for vegetarians. The quantities of each ingredient are listed, to show you how the daily nutritional analyses were calculated and also to give you an idea of how much food would be appropriate for young athletes. But it is not necessary to measure out their food so precisely every day! You may change the order of snacks and meals to suit individual training schedules. For more recipe ideas, *see* Chapter 6.

Menu for ... high-energy training (providing approximately 2500 calories)
Breakfast
Oatmeal made with 60 g oats, 300 ml skimmed milk, 1 tablespoon (20 g) of honey and 2 tablespoons (40 g) raisins

Snack
A serving (about 100 g) of fresh fruit
A granola bar

Lunch
Wholewheat roll filled with tuna (50 g), mayonnaise (1 tablespoon) and cucumber
2 containers (2 x 150 g) fruit yogurt
A serving (about 100 g) of fresh fruit

Pre-training snack (or afternoon snack)
A banana
A small handful (25 g) of nuts

During training
500 ml fruit juice mixed with 500 ml water

Post-training snack
300 ml flavored milk

Supper
Chicken and vegetable stir-fry (*see* recipe, page 120)
Boiled rice (85 g uncooked weight)

Nutrition
2550 kcal
116 g protein
66 g fat (17 g saturates)
398 g carbohydrate

Menu for ... high-energy training (providing approximately 3000 calories)

Breakfast
2 slices wholegrain toast with margarine (20 g) and 1 tablespoon (20 g) of honey
A serving (about 100 g) of fresh fruit

Snack
1 (80 g) home-made or ready-made pancake (*see* recipe for honey pancake, page 142)

Lunch
A wholewheat pita (75 g) filled with cooked turkey (130 g), salad and a tablespoon (20 g) of mayonnaise
Yogurt drink
A serving (about 100 g) of fresh fruit

Pre-training snack (or afternoon snack)
3 mini-pancakes with 1 tablespoon (20 g) of honey
A small handful of nuts (25 g)

During training
500 ml fruit juice mixed with 500 ml water

Post-training snack
A container of yogurt (150 g) and about 6 dried apricots (120 g)

Supper
2 generous slices of pizza (400 g; *see* recipe, page 123), with salad or vegetables
Rice pudding (170 g; ready made or home-made, *see* recipe page 139)

Nutrition
3058 kcal
123 g protein
90 g fat (26 g saturates)
468 g carbohydrate

Menu for ... high-energy training (providing approximately 3500 kcal)
Breakfast
2 poached eggs with 3 slices wholewheat toast and margarine (15 g)
A serving (about 100 g) of fresh fruit

Snack
A small handful of nuts (25 g) and raisins (60 g)

Lunch
2 wholewheat wraps filled with cooked chicken (80 g), 1 tablespoon (30 g)
mayonnaise and salad
A container (150 g) of fruit yogurt
A serving (about 100 g) of fresh fruit

Pre-training snack (or afternoon snack)
5 rice cakes with 1 tablespoon (30 g) peanut butter

During training
500 ml fruit juice diluted with 500 ml water

Post-training snack
300 ml semi-skimmed milk
2 granola bars

Supper
2 baked potatoes (400 g) with margarine (10 g)
Grilled haddock or other white fish (150 g) with vegetables or salad
2 bananas with a container (150 g) of fruit yogurt

Nutrition
3508 kcal
156 g protein
117 g fat (28 g saturates)
488 g carbohydrate

Menu for ... vegetarians

Breakfast
Oatmeal (70 g) and 300 ml skimmed milk, a sliced banana and a tablespoon (20 g) of honey
A serving (about 100 g) of fresh fruit

Snack
A handful of nuts (40 g) and about 6 (120 g) dried apricots

Lunch
Wholewheat pita bread (75 g) filled with 2 tablespoons (50 g) grated cheese, grated carrot and a little (20 g) mayonnaise
A container of yogurt (150 g)
Cherry tomatoes
A serving (about 100 g) of fresh fruit

Pre-training snack (or afternoon snack)
3 rice cakes with 1 tablespoon peanut butter

During training
500 ml fruit juice mixed with 500 ml water

Post-training snack
500 ml flavored milk or low-fat milkshake

Supper
Macaroni and cheese (200 g) with vegetables (*see* recipe, page 124)
A serving of strawberries or other fresh fruit (approx 100 g) with a container (150 g) of fruit yogurt

Nutrition
3048 kcal
115 g protein
99 g fat (28 g saturates)
453 g carbohydrate

References

ACSM, "Exercise and Fluid Replacement," *Medicine & Science in Sports & Exercise*, 39 (2007), pp. 377–390.

Betts, J. *et al.*, "The Influence of Carbohydrate and Protein Ingestion During Recovery from Prolonged Exercise on Subsequent Endurance Performance," *Journal of Sports Science*, 25(13) (2007), pp. 1449–1460.

Chryssanthopoulos, C. *et al.*, "The Effect of a High Carbohydrate Meal on Endurance Running Capacity," *International Journal of Sport Nutrition*, 12, (2002), pp. 157–71.

Cockburn, E. *et al.*, "Acute Milk-Based Protein-CHO Supplementation Attenuates Exercise-Induced Muscle Damage," *Applied Physiology, Nutrition, and Metabolism*, 33(4) (2008), pp. 775–783.

Coyle, E., "Fluid and Fuel Intake During Exercise," *Journal of Sports Science*, 22 (2004), pp. 39–55.

Gilson, S.F. *et al.*, "Effects of Chocolate Milk Consumption on Markers of Muscle Recovery During Intensified Soccer Training," *Medicine & Science in Sports & Exercise*, 41 (2009), p. S577

Gisolfi, C.V. *et al.*, "Effect of Sodium Concentration in a Carbohydrate-Electrolyte Solution on Intestinal Absorption," *Med. Sci. Sports Ex.*, 27(10) (1995), pp. 1414–1420.

Hargreaves, M. *et al.*, "Pre-Exercise Carbohydrate and Fat Ingestion: Effects on Metabolism and Performance," *Journal of Sports Science*, 22(1) (2004), pp. 31–38.

International Association of Athletic Federations (IAAF), *Nutrition for Athletics: The 2007 IAAF Consensus Statement* (IAAF, 2007).

International Olympic Committee (IOC), "Consensus on Sports Nutrition, 2003," *Journal of Sports Science*, 22(1) (2004), p. x.

Ivy, J.L. *et al.*, "Muscle Glycogen Synthesis After Exercise: Effect of Time of Carbohydrate Ingestion," *Journal of Applied Physiology*, 64 (1988), pp. 1480–1485.

Jeukendrup, A., "Carbohydrate Intake During Exercise and Performance," *Nutrition*, 20 (2004), pp. 669–677.

Kerksick, C. *et al.*, "International Society of Sports Nutrition Position Stand: Nutrient Timing," *Journal of the International Society of Sports Nutrition*, 3(5) (2008), p. 17.

Maughan, R.J. *et al.*, "Rehydration and Recovery After Exercise," *Sports Sci. Ex.*, 9(62) (1996), pp. 1–5.

Maughan, R.J. & Leiper, J.B., "Sodium intake and post-exercise rehydration in man," *European Journal of Applied Physiology*; 71(4):311-9.

National Federation of State High School Associations (NFSH), *Position Statement and Recommendations for the Use of Energy Drinks by Young Athletes* (NFSH, 2008).

Passe, D.H. *et al.*, "Palatability and Voluntary Intake of Sports Beverages, Diluted Orange Juice and Water During Exercise," *International Journal of Sport Nutrition and Exercise Metabolism*, 14 (2004), pp. 272–284.

Rodriquez, N.R., Di Marco, N.M. and Langley, S., "American College of Sports Medicine Position Stand: Nutrition and Athletic Performance. American Dietetic Association; Dietitians of Canada; American College of Sports Medicine," *Med Sci Sports Ex.*, 41(3) (2009), pp. 709–731.

Shireffs, S.M. *et al.*, "Milk as an Effective Post-Exercise Rehydration Drink," *British Journal of Nutrition*, 98 (2007), pp. 173–180.

Tarnopolsky, M. and MacLennan, D.P., "Post Exercise Protein-Carbohydrate and Carbohydrate Supplements Increase Muscle Glycogen in Males and Females," *Journal of Applied Physiology* (Abstracts), 4 (1997), p. 332A.

Van Loon, L.J.C., "Application of Protein or Protein Hydrolysates to Improve Post-exercise Recovery," *Applied Physiology, Nutrition, and Metabolism*, 17 (2007), pp. S104–117.

Zawadski, K.M. *et al.*, "Carbohydrate-protein complex increases the rate of muscle glycogen storage after exercise," *Journal of Applied Physiology* (1992), vol. 72, pp.1854-9.

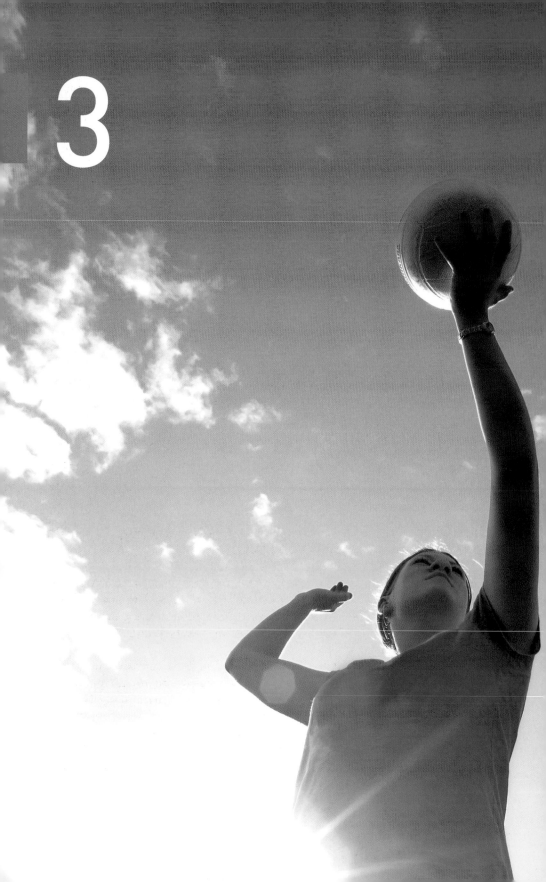

3

WEIGHT AND SPORTS PERFORMANCE

For many sports, a low body fat percentage is associated with improved performance, but for children and adolescents there is not necessarily a linear relationship between the two. The issue of body weight and body fat percentage should be treated sensitively as misguided remarks or advice to young athletes may inadvertently result in an unhealthy obsession about their weight, body shape and food generally.

Clearly, young athletes who are a healthy weight for their build should not be encouraged to lose weight. If they are unhappy about their weight, the problem may be one of low self-esteem or being ill matched to their sport. For example, children with a larger build would not be well matched to thin-build sports such as distance running, gymnastics or ballet dancing.

The question as to whether overweight young athletes should be encouraged to lose weight is a tricky one and this should be discussed with a health professional. Much depends on their age, development stage, current weight and motivating reasons for losing weight.

This chapter considers the implications of weight loss for young athletes. These can be both positive and negative, so it is essential that any decision to lose weight should be made with professional guidance. This chapter also provides sensible strategies for achieving weight loss as well as weight gain.

Is there a link between a young athlete's weight, body fat percentage and performance?

Leanness is generally associated with better performance for virtually all sports. Excess body fat hinders performance: it reduces speed, agility, balance and endurance. Even for activities where a high body weight is advantageous for generating momentum, such as throwing, those athletes with a higher lean body mass percentage and lower fat percentage perform better.

But it is crucial to understand that there is no "ideal" body fat percentage for young athletes. While improved performance is generally associated with lower-than-average body fat levels for many sports, there is certainly not a linear relationship between performance and body fat percentage. In other words, lower body fat levels are not always better. For each person, there is a range of body fat percentages at which they will perform at their best, and outside of which their performance and health are likely to suffer. Young athletes should not be put under pressure to attain an unrealistic low body weight and body fat percentage. Being lean does not guarantee athletic success.

Should overweight young athletes be encouraged to lose weight?

Any decision to lose weight should be made with the advice of a professional – such as a doctor, nutritionist or dietitian. Nutritional needs during this time are particularly high and important nutrients that are essential to children's health could be missed out.

Often, young athletes feel under pressure to lose weight to improve their performance and/or improve their appearance. They may see the successes of leaner competitors and be tempted to lose weight. Or they may feel frustrated by recent poor performance and perceive their weight to be the limiting factor for success in their sport. Sometimes, a decision to embark on a weight-loss regime may be triggered by a careless remark made by a well-meaning coach or teammate. The problem is that, without proper help, a desire to lose weight may develop into obsessive eating and exercise behavior that could put their performance and health at risk. In such cases, young athletes, whether overweight or not, should be discouraged from losing weight. Instead, parents and coaches should try to build the young athlete's self-esteem and help them feel more positive about their weight and performance. Praising their successes and emphasizing their strengths should help reduce undue anxiety about their weight.

On the other hand, for young athletes who are genuinely overweight, losing a few pounds through sensible eating and increased activity is likely to have a positive impact on their performance and health. It is important that they receive accurate information about nutrition, and positive support from their coach, family and friends.

How can I evaluate a young athlete's weight?

It can be difficult to evaluate whether young athletes have a weight problem. As a starting point, you can calculate their body mass index (BMI) – their weight in kg divided by the square of their height in meters – and compare with the children's BMI-for-age charts published by the US Centers for Disease Control and Prevention (CDC) (*see* http://www.cdc.gov/healthyweight/assessing/bmi/index.html). This will tell you whether their body weight is higher than average for their height and age. Table 3.1 gives the BMIs for overweight and obese children.

But BMI is not perfect. For example, it's very common for children to gain weight quickly – and for their BMI to go up – during puberty. They can also have a high BMI if they have a large frame or a lot of muscle, not excess fat. BMI does not differentiate between muscle and fat so it can be misleading when used with young athletes. Many of the world's top athletes have high BMIs due to their high muscularity, which would classify them as overweight. Thus, a young athlete who is relatively heavy due to a high muscle mass may have a high BMI for his or her age, and a child with a small frame may have a normal BMI but too much body fat.

It's important to look at the BMI values as a trend instead of focusing on individual numbers. Any one measurement, taken out of context, can give you the wrong impression of a young athlete's growth. The real value of BMI measurements lies in viewing them as a pattern over time. This allows doctors and parents to watch a child's growth and determine whether it is normal compared with that of other children of the same age.

To determine whether they have excess fat, further assessment would be needed. This might include bioelectrical impedance or skinfold thickness measurements.

Table 3.1 BMIs for overweight and obese children

Age	Overweight		Obese	
	Boys	Girls	Boys	Girls
5	17.4	17.1	19.3	19.2
6	17.6	17.3	19.8	19.7
7	17.9	17.8	20.6	20.5
8	18.4	18.3	21.6	21.6
9	19.1	19.1	22.8	22.8
10	19.8	19.9	24.0	24.1
11	20.6	20.7	25.1	25.4
12	21.2	21.7	26.0	26.7
13	21.9	22.6	26.8	27.8

Source: Cole *et al.* (2000)

How can I measure body fat percentage in young athletes?

Body fat levels in children and adolescents can be estimated using bioelectrical impedance or skinfold thickness measurements.

Bioelectrical impedance

This is the principle used in body composition analyzers and body fat scales, widely available in shops and gyms. Many are calibrated for different ages and both genders, and are suitable for use with young athletes (Phillips *et al.*, 2003). A mild electrical current (completely painless!) is sent through the body, either from foot to foot or foot to opposite hand. The current passes more easily and more quickly through lean mass, but much more slowly through fat mass. The more body fat present, the greater the resistance. This method is less accurate for very lean and very overweight people.

Skinfold thickness

This method is widely used in sports clubs and has been shown to provide an accurate estimate of body fat percentage in children and adolescents (Deurenberg, 1990). The callipers measure the thickness of the layer of fat beneath the skin at various sites of the body. It works on the theory that 50 percent of the total body fat is stored under the skin. Most assessments involve measurements at four sites: the triceps, biceps, below the shoulder blades, and midway between the hip and navel. The accuracy depends on the level of skill of the person taking the measurements. It is less accurate for very lean and obese individuals.

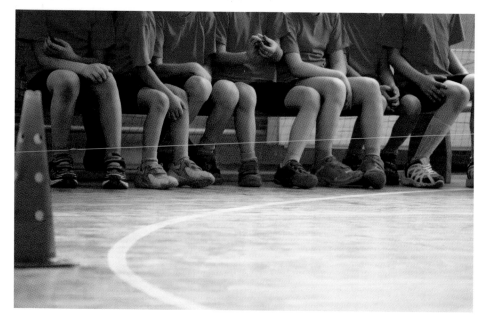

Figures 3.1 and 3.2 show the body fat ranges for males and females aged 4–20 years that would be classified as under-fat, healthy, over-fat and obese (Jebb *et al.*, 2004).

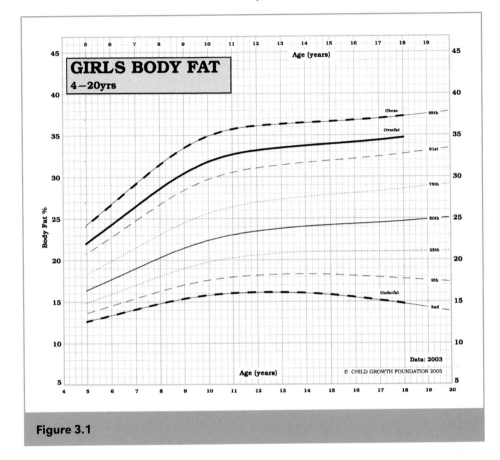

Figure 3.1

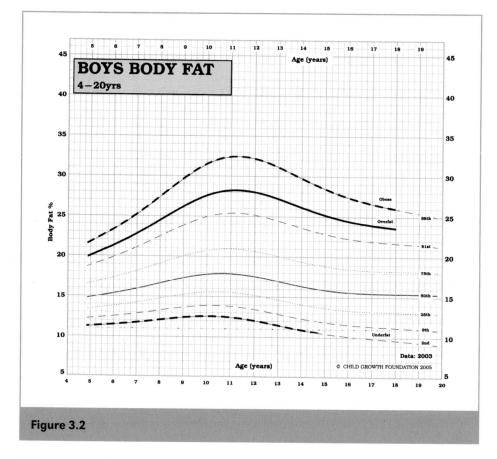

Figure 3.2

What are the next steps?

If you think a young athlete has gained too much weight or is too thin, you should consult a doctor, nutritionist, dietitian or other health professional to help you decide whether they really have a weight problem. They may ask questions about the athlete's health, level of physical activity and eating habits, as well as family medical history. They can put all this information together to determine whether there is a weight or growth problem.

If your adviser thinks the athlete's weight isn't in the healthy range, they should provide specific dietary and exercise recommendations. For children and teenagers, significantly restricting calories or following fad diets or starvation plans can deprive them of the nutrients their growing bodies need, and may actually slow down growth and development.

What's a healthy weight loss strategy for young athletes?

It is important that any weight loss goal is realistic and achievable for the young athlete's build and level of maturity. You should discourage strict dieting, diuretics (substances that cause the body to lose water through urination), excessive exercise and the use of saunas as weight-loss methods, as these can be very dangerous for young athletes. In the short term, these methods may result in dehydration, low muscle glycogen stores, fatigue and poor performance. In the long term, they may lead to a repetitive cycle of weight loss and gain (yo-yo dieting), food or weight obsession, or disordered eating.

For most young athletes, the best thing you can do is to encourage a balanced diet and regular physical activity. Talk to them about healthy eating and exercise, teach by example and let them make their own decisions about food. Don't put them on a "diet." Instead make healthy changes to what they eat.

But, for competitive athletes who need to reduce their body fat in order to get to the next competitive level, the off-season or holidays is the best time to do it. During this time, they will be able to cut calories and lose weight sensibly without it having a negative effect on their performance or health.

If they try to lose weight in season, they risk poor performance because the combination of strenuous training and cutting calories places a lot of stress on the body. They won't be able to train hard day after day on too few calories. Cutting calories means that they will not get enough carbohydrates to replenish their muscle fuel stores. This can lead to chronic fatigue, muscle loss and under-performance. Too few calories in combination with an intense training schedule can also reduce immunity and leave them susceptible to illnesses.

Build self-esteem

If you can build young athletes' self-esteem and help them feel more positive about themselves they are more likely to make healthier food choices. Make a point of praising their accomplishments, emphasize their strengths and encourage them to try new skills to foster success. Don't tell a young athlete that they are "greedy" or "lazy." Do tell them that you recognize how hard it is to make healthy choices at times. Never call them fat or tell them to lose weight. Let them know that it is what's inside that matters, and play down your concerns about their weight – or even your own weight.

Set a good example

Young athletes are more likely to copy what their parents do than what they say. They learn a lot about food and activity by watching their parents. They should see that you exercise and eat a balanced diet. Share mealtimes as often as possible and eat the same meals. Don't make a young athlete feel guilty about their eating habits. Do praise them when you see them eating healthily.

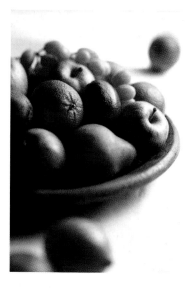

Don't use food as a reward

Rewarding good behavior with sweet treats only reinforces the idea that they are a special treat and makes children crave them more. Allow them in moderation – say, on one day of the week and at the end of a meal.

Don't ban any foods

Banning a food increases a young athlete's desire for it and makes it more likely that they will eat it in secret. Allow all foods but explain that certain ones should be eaten only now and then or kept as occasional treats. If they know that they can eat a little of their favorite food every day, they will stop thinking of it as a forbidden food and then won't want to binge on it.

Provide healthy snacks

Instead of cookies, chips and chocolate, make sure there are healthier alternatives onhand. Fresh fruit, low-fat yogurt, wholewheat toast and wholegrain breakfast cereals are good choices.

HEALTHY SNACKS FOR A HEALTHY WEIGHT

- Fresh fruit
- Wholewheat toast
- Low-fat yogurt
- Low-fat milk
- A few nuts or seeds
- Wholegrain breakfast cereal with milk
- Vegetable crudités (carrot, peppers and cucumber sticks)
- Granola bar
- Rice cakes

Get them moving more

Although young athletes train and play sport, they may be quite inactive the rest of the time. Look for opportunities to increase their daily activity. For example, encourage them to walk or cycle to and from school. Try to increase the amount of exercise you do together as a family – swimming, playing football, a family walk or bike ride.

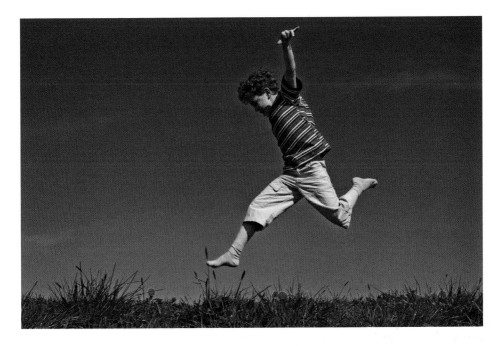

Don't snack-and-view

Discourage eating meals or unhealthy snacks while watching television. Because their mind will be on the television and not on the food, they won't notice when they are full up or not hungry any more.

Top tips for maintaining a healthy weight

The following strategies will make it easier for young athletes to achieve a healthy weight.

- They should eat foods that fill them up, not out – starting a meal with a bowl of soup, a salad, some fresh fruit or some fresh vegetables helps take the edge of hunger pangs. People who follow this eating pattern feel more satisfied at the end of a meal and consume fewer calories.
- Ditch the fizz – drinking water rather than sugary carbonated drinks is a good way of saving calories, and water won't rot their teeth or leach calcium from their bones.
- Follow the one-third rule – vegetables or salad should fill at least one-third of the plate. This will help satisfy hunger as well as providing essential nutrients.
- They should always eat food sitting at a table – eating in front of the TV or eating on the run makes people eat more because they don't concentrate fully.

- They should never skip meals – no matter how busy they are. Leaving gaps longer than four hours between meals not only saps energy but also triggers muscle loss, as the body turns to protein for fuel. Young athletes should eat three small meals spread over the day – breakfast, lunch and evening meal – with two healthy snacks in between. Small, regular meals keep the metabolism revved up so that more calories are burned off each day.
- Replace full-fat dairy products with low-fat varieties – they contain just as much protein and calcium.
- They should opt for brown instead of white – wholegrain bread, bran cereals and whole-wheat pasta are rich in fiber, which will make them feel fuller. They should make the switch gradually, though, to avoid stomach upsets.
- Make sure they don't wolf down their food – eating food slowly and in a relaxed state of mind will curb the desire to eat more then they need. According to research, scoffing a meal means that the satiety center in the brain doesn't receive the right signals, and explains why people may eat more than they need.
- They should start the day with a healthy breakfast, such as oatmeal. People who skip breakfast to "save calories" are more likely to overeat later in the day and pile on unwanted pounds.
- Get them to eat until they are satisfied, not stuffed. They should eat when they are truly hungry and stop when they feel satisfied, and avoid eating to the point where they feel stuffed and uncomfortable. By eating a bit slower, the brain has more time to get the "full up" message.
- They should avoid mindless munching – help them to find another distraction, or eat something that's low in calories, such as carrot sticks or apple slices.

Can young athletes be too thin?

If you are worried about a young athlete being too thin, it's important to understand that many children who weigh less than others their age are perfectly healthy. They may go through puberty later than some of their peers, and their bodies may grow and change at a different rate. Most underweight teens catch up in weight as they finish puberty during their later teen years, and there's rarely a need to try to gain weight.

In a few cases, young athletes can be underweight because of a health problem. If they feel tired or are ill frequently, or have symptoms such as a cough, stomach ache, diarrhea or other problems that have lasted for more than a week or two, seek the advice of your doctor.

Some young athletes are underweight because of eating disorders, like anorexia or bulimia, that require attention. The pressure to be thin or attain better performance may trigger unhealthy eating behaviors that put their health at risk. It has been estimated that up to 60 percent of female athletes suffer from disordered eating (Sundgot-Borgen, 1994). It appears to be more common in athletes involved in "thin-build" sports, where a low body weight, low body fat percentage or thin build is perceived to be advantageous (Beals and Manore, 2002). These can be considered in four categories, as shown in Table 3.2.

According to a 2001 study at the University of Leeds, UK, 16 percent of elite female middle- and long-distance runners had anorexia or bulimia, compared with 1–2 percent of the general population (Hulley and Hill, 2001). A 2004 study of 1620 male and female elite Norwegian athletes found that 42 percent of women competing in aesthetic sports and 24 percent of those competing in endurance events met the clinical criteria for an eating disorder (Sundgot-Borgen and Torstveit, 2004).

Table 3.2 High-risk sports for eating disorders

Aesthetic sports	Endurance sports and low-weight performance sports	Weight-division sports	Gym sports
Gymnastics	Middle-distance and long-distance running	Lightweight rowing	Bodybuilding
Figure skating	Cycling	Judo	Aerobics
Ballet and dance	Swimming	Karate	Fitness
Synchronized swimming	Horse racing	Wrestling	
		Boxing	

What are eating disorders?

Eating disorders are serious psychiatric illnesses that require medical, psychiatric or behavioral treatments. The two most well-recognized forms are anorexia nervosa and bulimia nervosa. Anorexia nervosa is an extremely restrictive eating behavior in which the individual continues to restrict food and feel fat in spite of being 15 percent or more below an ideal body weight. Bulimia nervosa refers to a cycle of food restriction followed by bingeing and purging.

Disordered eating is a general term used to describe a wide range of abnormal and harmful eating behaviors that sufferers use to try to lose weight or maintain an abnormally low body weight. These may include limiting certain foods or food groups, severely restricting calorie intake, or occasional bingeing and purging.

What are the symptoms of anorexia?
According to the American Psychiatric Association's (APA) *Diagnostic and Statistical Manual of Mental Disorders* (DSM-IV) criteria, anorexia nervosa is diagnosed in a person who:

- weighs at least 15 percent less than the minimum average for his or her height but has no physical illness causing the weight loss;
- has an intense fear of gaining weight or "becoming fat";
- has severe body dissatisfaction, sees her/himself as "fat" despite being underweight;
- is suffering from amenorrhea (absence of at three consecutive periods).

Sufferers are in continual pursuit of thinness and try to achieve this through self-starvation. Many anorexics exercise excessively to burn off extra calories and avoid fatness. The characteristics and warning signs of anorexia are summarized in Table 3.3.

Table 3.3 Characteristics and warning signs of anorexia nervosa

Characteristics	Warning signs
Weight 15% lower than minimum average for height	Excessive loss of weight
Self-starvation	Feel fat even when thinner than other athletes
Obsessive fear of weight gain	Often lie to family and friends about what they have eaten
Feeling fat when thin	Constantly think about weight loss and food
Low self-esteem	Periods have stopped, or never started
Social withdrawal	Frequent weighing
Distorted body image	Difficulty sleeping
Obsessive exercise	Layer of soft hair over the body

What are the symptoms of bulimia?

People with bulimia nervosa tend to use extreme methods to lose weight, alternating between strict dieting and overeating. The main features of bulimia nervosa as defined by the DSM-IV criteria are:

- episodes of binge eating followed by purging that have occurred at least twice a week for three months;
- feeling out of control during the bingeing and purging episodes;
- being dissatisfied with your body image.

After a binge, people with bulimia feel guilt, shame and anxiety, and will then try to purge their body of the food by vomiting, exercising excessively, or using laxatives or diuretics. The characteristics and warning signs of bulimia are summarized in Table 3.4.

Table 3.4 Characteristics and warning signs of bulimia nervosa

Characteristics	Warning signs
Bingeing on large amounts of food	Regularly suffers from sore throats and experiences infections
Guilt and remorse after bingeing	Face appears puffy or swollen
Purging	Periods are irregular
Starvation	Obsessed with losing weight
Excessive exercise	Self-induced vomiting after meals or taking laxatives to lose weight
Distorted body image	Eating in secret, lying to family and friends about eating habits
Obsession with food and weight	Emotional and depressed, mood swings

What causes eating disorders in young athletes?

There is no single cause of eating disorders or disordered eating in young athletes but it often stems from a belief that a lower body weight enhances athletic success. The athlete begins to diet and, for reasons not completely understood, then adopts more restrictive and unhealthy eating behaviors. The pressures or demands of certain sports or training programs, or the requests made by coaches to lose weight may trigger an eating disorder in susceptible individuals.

Sometimes a negative comment about the athlete's weight from a coach or teammate can trigger disordered eating, particularly in adolescents, who are more vulnerable to the negative opinions of their peers and eager to feel accepted by them.

It's possible that the young athlete's personality may put them at greater risk than a non-athlete for developing disordered eating. Successful athletes tend to be highly driven, perfectionist, self-motivated, competitive and goal-orientated – the same traits seen in people with eating disorders.

THE EATING DISORDERS "PERSONALITY"

- Low self-esteem
- Perfectionism
- Tenacity or obsessiveness
- High need for approval
- High achieving
- Competitiveness

What are the warning signs for eating disorders?

Look out for the following warning signs and types of behavior that could indicate an eating problem in young athletes.

- Unexplained losses in performance
- An obsession with body image, shape and weight
- Constant use of weighing scales
- Missing meals or avoiding certain foods
- An obsession with quantities or proportions of food in the diet
- Rapid mood swings
- Rapid and significant weight loss

What are the effects of eating disorders on health and performance?

Young athletes with disordered eating and eating disorders are likely to develop health problems, nutritional deficiencies, chronic fatigue and dehydration, and to experience a dramatic reduction in performance.

Health problems

For females, severe food restriction and dramatic weight loss, particularly when combined with intense exercise, lead to disturbances in the menstrual cycle – menstrual dysfunction. Menstrual periods can become irregular (oligomenorrhea) or stop altogether (amenorrhea). Without enough estrogen to maintain and increase bone mass, the bones get weaker, more porous and lighter. This may result in osteopenia, a lower-than-normal bone density, or premature osteoporosis, a more severe loss of bone mineral density.

A young athlete with menstrual dysfunction should be encouraged to increase her energy intake and modify her exercise program. Experts advise lowering the intensity and volume of training by 10–15 percent, including phases of lower-intensity training or rest, and eating a little more. Studies are ongoing to determine just how many calories are needed for normal menses to resume, but so far it appears that even small increases in body weight (1–3 kg) may be all that is required to resume normal menstrual cycles by reversing the negative energy balance that caused the problem.

HEALTH CONSEQUENCES OF EATING DISORDERS

- Amenorrhea (cessation of periods) and infertility
- Heart problems, such as abnormal heart rhythm, low blood pressure and cardiac failure
- Osteoporosis, weakened bones, risk of fracture
- Erosion of dental enamel
- Gastrointestinal problems such as peptic ulcers
- Kidney problems
- Low white blood cell count and poor immunity
- Metabolic problems
- Difficulty maintaining body temperature

Effect on performance

Ironically, in the short term, there may be an improvement, rather than a drop, in performance. Many athletes with eating disorders use stimulants such as caffeine or diet pills to suppress their appetite and maintain their energy. But, eventually, restrictive eating rebounds on health and performance will suffer. As glycogen and nutrient stores become chronically depleted, the athlete's health will suffer and optimal performance cannot be sustained indefinitely. Low glycogen stores result in increased fatigue and reduced performance. Without enough protein to maintain and repair muscle, there will be a loss of lean body mass, strength and endurance. The athlete quickly becomes more susceptible to injury, illness and infection. Deficiencies of vitamins and minerals will eventually develop, and these will affect performance too, increasing the risk of muscle weakness, injuries and infections.

How should I help a young athlete with an eating disorder?

Eating disorders are illnesses that require proper treatment. If you suspect a young athlete of having an eating disorder, here are some ways you can help.

- Plan the conversation for a quiet time and place.
- Think about what you will say in advance.
- Be tactful, tread very gently and avoid accusations.

- Do not present "evidence,"confront them with accusations or try to "catch them out" to prove your case.
- Don't make demands such as "Stop doing this to yourself."
- Just state your concern and your wish for them to seek help.
- Don't try to cure their behavior or give solutions – they need proper help from an expert.
- Have an eating disorders hotline number, website details, brochure or book with you.

What treatment is available?

Various forms of specialist help are available, including trained counselors from a self-help organization or a private eating disorders clinic. A doctor can provide a referral for treatment with a multidisciplinary team of psychologists and dietitians. This may be within a hospital or clinic. Bear in mind, though, that even when eating disorders are identified, treatment can take many months or years. Doctors, therapists, supportive family and teammates can help athletes learn new ways of thinking and feeling about how they eat, why they train and what it means to be healthy.

The ultimate goal of treatment is to normalize weight and eating behavior, and to deal with the psychological issues that lie behind the eating disorder. Whatever form of help the athlete chooses, the support of friends and family is very important.

Can eating disorders be prevented?

With young athletes, always emphasize that nutrition is fundamental to good performance. Stress the importance of food as fuel – not just something that determines body size. Help young athletes understand that if they have too low a calorie intake this will reduce their performance and muscle strength.

If they feel pressured to lose weight, encourage them to speak to their coach and seek advice from a registered nutritionist or dietitian. Make sure they don't cut out food groups or impose strict food rules (e.g. no fat, no "junk" food) – they need to choose a wide variety of different foods to get their daily intake of nutrients. Overly strict rules can sometimes result in obsessive eating behavior. Discourage dieting, particularly quick-fix and fad diets that don't provide enough energy to support a training program.

PREVENTING AND DEALING WITH EATING DISORDERS

- Young athletes should be realistic about their goal weight – they may be striving to attain a weight lower than is appropriate for their genetic body type.
- If they have weight to lose, ensure that they don't crash-diet. Seek advice from a nutritionist or dietitian if you are struggling to help them balance food intake and exercise.
- Aim to help them eat a balanced diet, including a wide variety of foods from each food group (*see* Chapter 1) and adequate calcium to maintain bone density. Include three to four servings of dairy products or other calcium-rich foods daily (*see* page 37).
- If a young female athlete has suffered amenorrhea for longer than six months, she should seek advice from her GP, to rule out medical causes of amenorrhea.
- If her periods stop or become irregular, her training frequency, volume and intensity should be reduced, or her current program should be changed.
- If a young athlete suffers from disordered eating, they will need help in overcoming this problem (*see* page 75).

Weight gain

What can young athletes eat to gain weight?

Many young athletes struggle to keep up their weight or put on any weight, because they burn a lot of energy in sport. However, only after puberty should young athletes attempt to add muscle bulk. In the meantime, the goal should be to combine their normal training with an eating plan that provides sufficient energy and nutrients to meet their needs. Their daily energy requirement will be considerably higher than that of their non-active peers, which means they may find it difficult to consume enough food to satisfy their needs. Encourage them to eat more frequent meals and snacks, say, three meals and three or four healthy snacks in between. Make the energy and nutrient content of the food more concentrated. Here are some suggestions.

- Serve bigger portions, particularly of pasta, potatoes, rice, cereals, dairy products and protein-rich foods.
- Provide three to four nutritious snacks between meals (*see* the box entitled "High energy snacks for weight gain" for suggestions).
- Provide nutritious drinks (e.g. milk, flavored milk, hot chocolate, home-made milkshakes, yogurt drinks, fruit smoothies and fruit juice).
- Add grated cheese to vegetables, soups, potatoes, pasta dishes and stews.
- Add dried fruit to breakfast cereals, oatmeal and yogurt.

- Spread bread, toast or crackers with nutrient-dense spreads such as peanut butter and hummus.
- Serve vegetables and main courses with a nutritious sauce, such as cheese sauce.
- Instead of filling up with "junk," supplement their diet with high-energy, nutritious foods such as milk, nuts and dried fruits.
- Boost meals with healthy puddings, e.g. rice pudding, banana custard, fruit crumble with yogurt, yogurt or custard mixed with fruit, bread pudding and pancakes.

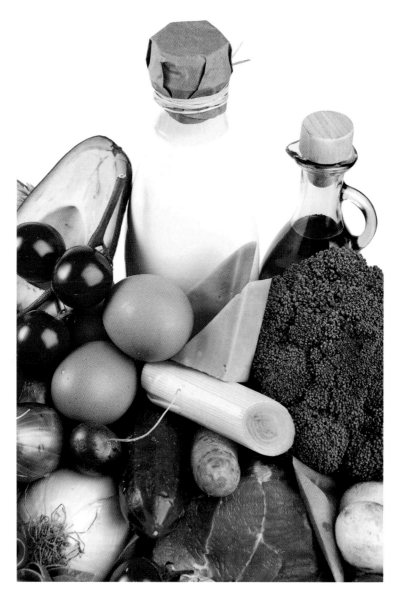

How can young athletes increase muscle mass?
Training

To add muscle mass, their muscles need a stimulus to get bigger and stronger, and that requires a well-designed resistance training program. Previous beliefs that resistance training can damage the growth cartilage or stunt their growth have proven to be unfounded – there have been no cases of bone damage in relation to resistance training. Exercises that emphasize strengthening of the core are recommended for pre-adolescent and adolescent children. Only after they have passed puberty should they consider adding muscle bulk. The best guidance comes from the American Academy of Paediatrics Committee on Sports Medicine and Fitness. Here is a summary of its updated policy statement (American Academy of Pediatrics, 2008):

- *Strength training programs for pre-adolescents and adolescents can be safe and effective if proper resistance training techniques and safety precautions are followed.*
- *Pre-adolescents and adolescents should avoid competitive weight lifting, power lifting, body building, and maximal lifts until they reach physical and skeletal maturity.*
- *Before beginning a formal strength training program, a medical evaluation should be performed. If indicated, a referral may be made to a sports medicine specialist who is familiar with various strength training methods as well as risks and benefits in pre-adolescents and adolescents.*
- *Aerobic conditioning should be coupled with resistance training if general health benefits are the goal.*
- *Strength training programs should include a warm-up and cool-down component.*
- *Specific strength training exercises should be learned initially with no load (resistance). Once the exercise skill has been mastered, incremental loads can be added.*
- *Progressive resistance exercise requires the successful completion of 8 to 15 repetitions in good form before increasing weight or resistance.*
- *A general strengthening program should address all major muscle groups and exercise through the complete range of motion.*
- *Any sign of injury or illness from strength training should be evaluated before continuing the exercise in question.*

Nutrition

The nutritional part of the equation for adding muscle mass is consuming adequate energy and nutrients, with energy perhaps being the most important. When it comes to adding muscle, many young (and also adult) athletes make the mistake of focusing solely on protein intake. To put on muscle, they need to consume about 500 more calories than they burn each day. They do need a little extra protein but most can get this from a balanced diet. In fact, the timing of their protein intake in relation to workouts is just as important as the amount.

Resistance training increases the rate at which muscle protein is made after a training session. So encourage young athletes to consume around 10–20 g protein within 30 minutes of training and as part of their protein–carbohydrate recovery snack (*see* Chapter 2, page 55, "What should young athletes eat after training?"). This will help repair muscle tissue damaged during training, and support the making of new muscle tissue proteins. The meal or snack should contain about four times as much carbohydrate as protein. Good options include low-fat milk, flavoured milk, yogurt, yogurt drinks or home-made milkshakes (*see* page 57, "Refuelling snacks and drinks").

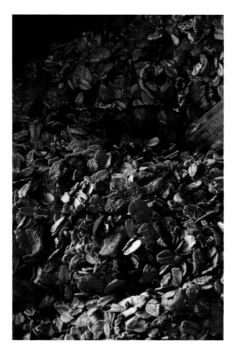

HIGH-ENERGY SNACKS FOR WEIGHT GAIN

- Nuts – peanuts, almonds, cashews, brazilnuts, pistachios
- Dried fruit – raisins, apricots, dates
- Sandwiches, rolls, wraps and bagels filled with cheese, chicken, ham, tuna, peanut butter or banana
- Yogurt
- Milk, milkshakes, flavored milk, yogurt drinks
- Breakfast cereal or oatmeal with milk
- Cheese
- Grilled cheese
- Mini-pancakes, scones, fruit muffins, banana bread
- Granola bars
- Bread or toast with jam or honey

References

American Academy of Pediatrics, "Strength Training by Children and Adolescents," *Pediatrics*, 121(4) (2008), pp. 835–840.

Beals, K.A. and Manore, M.M., "Disorders of the Female Athlete Triad Among Collegiate Athletes," *International Journal of Sport Nutrition and Exercise Metabolism*, 12 (2002), pp. 281–293.

Cole, T.J., Bellizzi, M., Flegal, K. and Dietz, W.H., "Establishing a Standard Definition for Child Overweight and Obesity Worldwide: International Survey," *British Medical Journal*, 320 (2000), pp. 1240–1243.

Deurenberg, P., "The Assessment of the Body Fat Percentage by Skinfold Thickness Measurements in Childhood and Young Adolescence," *British Journal of Nutrition*, 63 (1990), pp. 293–303.

Hulley, A.J. and Hill, A.J. "Eating Disorders and Health in Elite Women Distance Runners," *International Journal of Eating Disorders*, 30(3) (2001), pp. 312–317.

Jebb, S., McCarthy, D., Fry, T. and Prentice, A.M., "New Body Fat Reference Curves for Children," *Obesity Reviews* (NAASO suppl.) (2004), p. A146.

Phillips, S.M., Bandini, L.G., Compton, D.V., Naumova, E.N. and Must, A.A., "Longitudinal Comparison of Body Composition by Total Body Water and Bioelectrical Impedance in Adolescent Girls," *Journal of Nutrition*, 133(5) (1 May, 2003), pp. 1419–1425.

Sundgot-Borgen, J., "Eating Disorders in Female Athletes," *Sports Medicine*, 17(3) (1994), pp. 176–188.

Sundgot-Borgen, J. and Torstveit, M.K., "Prevalence of Eating Disorders in Elite Athletes is Higher than in the General Population," *Clinical Journal of Sport Medicine*, 14(1) (2004), pp. 25–32.

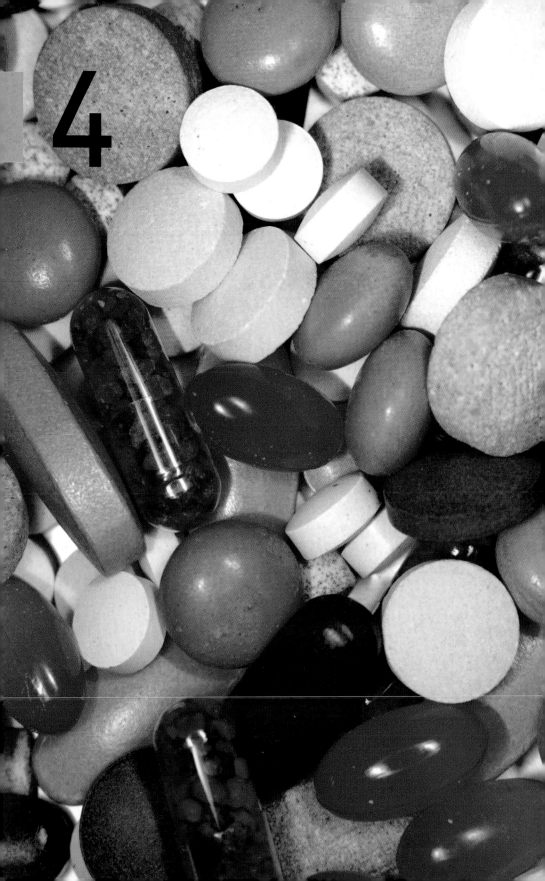

4

NUTRITIONAL SUPPLEMENTS

In the quest to improve their performance and gain a competitive edge, many young athletes take nutritional supplements, often without really knowing what they are or how they work. A 2005 survey revealed that 62 percent of UK junior national track and field athletes used them regularly (Nieper, 2005). Each athlete took an average of 2.4 supplements. Multivitamins and minerals were the most popular, but 17 different supplements were identified in the survey. In another study of adolescent German athletes, 80 percent reported taking various supplements, including sports drinks and energy supplements (Braun *et al.*, 2009).

So do young athletes really need them? Are they likely to benefit or harm their performance? The fact that many adult athletes take supplements does not mean that they are safe or effective for children and adolescents. Currently, nutritional supplements are not regulated for safety, purity, potency or efficacy, and manufacturers do not have to demonstrate that they are safe for children. Supplements may contain impurities or interact with medicines, and there is a possibility that certain products may contain impurities that would cause a positive drugs test (Schänzer, 2002).

This chapter provides information and evidence about the most popular nutritional supplements, to help you make up your own mind.

Caffeine

Young athletes often take caffeine in the form of energy drinks, sports drinks or cola before and during training or competition, in the belief that it will enhance their endurance, performance, concentration, motivation and mental alertness, and mask fatigue.

So what exactly is caffeine? It is a stimulant and, strictly speaking, is classed as a drug rather than a nutritional supplement. It is found in many everyday drinks, such as coffee, black and green tea, and cola, as well as chocolate (cocoa), and some brands of sports drinks, energy drinks and gels.

Caffeine works by decreasing the perception of effort during exercise, therefore allowing the athlete to perform at a higher intensity. It boosts adrenaline levels, which increases the levels of fatty acids in the bloodstream and encourages the muscles to use more fatty acids instead of glucose or glycogen (carbohydrate) for fuel. In theory, at least, caffeine may help athletes exercise longer and harder.

There are no official UK guidelines on caffeine for children but a review undertaken by Health Canada scientists considers 85 mg per day safe for 10–12 year olds

(Health and Welfare Canada, 2003). Food Standards Australia New Zealand recommends that children consume less than 95 mg per day (FSANZ, 2000). High doses of caffeine (greater than 95 mg daily) greatly increase the risks of negative side-effects – nervousness, an upset stomach, difficulty sleeping, anxiety, rapid heartbeat, dizziness and headaches – in some individuals. This equates to a cup of coffee, two cups of tea, or approximately one (500 ml) caffeinated sports drink or one (250 ml) energy drink.

But the safety and effectiveness of consuming caffeine before and during exercise has yet to be established with children and teenage athletes. They may be extra sensitive to caffeine so could experience the negative side-effects more than adults and end up suffering from "caffeine jitters" at a time when they are already nervous and anxious. The side-effects may outweigh the potential benefits of caffeine for performance.

It's also worth remembering that caffeine is a diuretic, which means that it causes the body to lose water through urination. While studies with adults suggest that regular, moderate caffeine intakes do not dehydrate the body, the effect of caffeinated sports drinks on hydration in young athletes remains unknown. High doses – equivalent to one or two sports drinks – or infrequent caffeine consumption may have a more noticeable diuretic effect in young athletes.

The bottom line is that there are still many unknowns about the effect of caffeine on the performance and health of young athletes. Until more research is done, caffeine cannot be recommended.

THE CAFFEINE CONTENT OF VARIOUS FOODS AND DRINKS

- Instant coffee – 60 mg/cup
- Espresso – 100 mg/shot
- Filter – 120 mg/cup
- Tea – 40 mg/cup
- Green tea – 40 mg/cup
- Sports drinks with caffeine (e.g. Powerade Energy) – 32 mg/100 ml
- Energy drinks (e.g. Red Bull) – 80 mg/250 ml
- Cola – 40 mg/330 ml
- Energy gel – 25 mg/sachet
- Dark chocolate – 40 mg/50 g
- Milk chocolate – 12 mg/50 g

Creatine

Creatine is extremely popular with adult athletes, who use it for its purported performance-boosting and muscle-building effects. Although the use of creatine is not recommended in people less than 18 years of age, several reports indicate widespread use in young athletes (Metzi *et al.*, 2001).

Creatine is a protein that is made naturally in the body from three amino acids, but can also be found in meat and fish, or taken in higher doses as a supplement. It is most commonly taken as a powder mixed with water or within an "all-in-one" protein and energy mix.

In the body it combines with phosphorus to form phosphocreatine (PC) in the muscle cells. This is an energy-rich compound that fuels the muscles during anaerobic activities, such as lifting weights, sprinting, jumping or throwing. The aim of creatine supplementation is to enhance the muscles' content of PC, which in turn would increase the amount of energy generated during brief periods of high-intensity exercise. Theoretically, it may allow athletes to sustain all-out effort longer than usual, recover faster between "sets" of high-intensity exercise, and increase muscle mass and strength gains. Indeed, studies with adult athletes have suggested that creatine supplements can improve performance in high-intensity activities, as well as increase total and lean body weight (Volek and Kraemer, 1996). However, there have been some studies showing no effect of creatine supplementation on performance (Kreider, 2003). It doesn't work for some individuals and is also unlikely to benefit endurance performance.

Unfortunately, there is little information about creatine use or the potential health risk in children and adolescents. Whether it is effective or safe in the long term has not been established. It is worth considering that performance during childhood and adolescence tends to be limited by mechanical factors rather than the relative contribution of the aerobic and anaerobic energy systems. A review by US researchers published in the *Journal of Strength and Conditioning Research* concluded that there is not enough research to support the use of creatine supplements by children and adolescents (Unnithan *et al.*, 2001).

Until the safety of creatine can be established in adolescents, the use of this product should be discouraged.

Energy bars

Energy bars are rich in carbohydrates and claim to provide a good source of fuel before and during exercise. However, don't assume that they will make anyone feel more energetic – that's what the manufacturers would want you to believe! The name on the label actually refers to the bar's high energy (calorie) content per gram.

The main ingredients are sugars (glucose, corn syrup, fructose) and maltodextrins (a carbohydrate made from corn starch). Bars may also contain small amounts of soy or whey protein, oat bran or cereal. Typically, they provide between 200 and 250 calories and 40–45 g of carbohydrate per bar. The protein and fat content is usually low.

On the plus side, consuming an energy bar before exercise may help increase endurance and improve performance – but not necessarily more than other carbohydrate-rich foods. Manufacturers also claim that energy bars provide a sustained source of energy, due to their high content of maltodextrin, which is digested more slowly than sugars. This results in a slower increase in blood sugar levels, compared with glucose (i.e. a low glycaemic response), which studies suggest can help increase endurance performance (Thomas *et al.*, 1991). But other foods can provide a similar performance benefit. Suitable pre-exercise snacks include cereal bars, dried fruit, bananas, and rice cakes with peanut butter.

On the minus side, the cost of energy bars may be prohibitive for young athletes. Explain to them that energy bars are not necessarily better for their performance than other foods, that they can get similar benefits from cheaper foods. Be aware, too, of the energy (calorie) content of bars. Many brands contain the same number of calories as popular chocolate and confectionery bars, and may be more than the athlete is likely to burn during the activity session! Over-consuming calories may result in weight gain.

In conclusion, the main benefit of consuming an energy bar before or during exercise is convenience. They are portable and non-perishable but there is no reason why they represent a better snack option than other high-carbohydrate foods.

Energy gels

Energy gels are carbohydrate-rich, jelly-like supplements that come in small squeezy sachets and are designed to be consumed on the move during endurance exercise. Many athletes appreciate their convenience but you should also be aware of alternative ways of fueling on the go.

Energy gels consist almost entirely of simple sugars (such as fructose and glucose) and maltodextrin (made from corn starch). Some brands also contain sodium, potassium and caffeine (*see* the section on caffeine, above). Most contain between 18 and 25 g of carbohydrate per sachet.

On the plus side, gels provide a convenient way of consuming carbohydrate during intense endurance exercise lasting longer than an hour. Their small size means that they can easily be stashed in pockets, opened with ease when running, for example, and consumed quickly in the manner of knocking back a "shot." They provide around 18–25 g of rapidly absorbed carbohydrate, which should fuel between 30 and 60 minutes of exercise. The scientific consensus is to consume 30–60 g of carbohydrate per hour during prolonged exercise in order to delay fatigue and improve endurance (Rodriquez *et al.*, 2009).

On the downside, some people dislike their texture, sweetness and intensity of flavor – it's really down to personal preference. Gels don't provide hydration so, if young athletes want to use them, encourage them to drink plenty of water at the same time. A handy rule of thumb would be to follow one sachet with 500 ml of water consumed over 60 minutes, or half a gel sachet followed by 250 ml of water over 30 minutes. If they don't drink enough, they could end up with stomach ache as the gel sits in their stomach. Drinking plenty of water effectively dilutes the gel, allowing the carbohydrate to be absorbed quickly into the bloodstream. In the same way as for energy bars, don't assume that energy gels will make athletes feel more energetic – they simply provide energy in a concentrated form.

In conclusion, energy gels provide convenient refueling during long, hard training sessions lasting longer than an hour, but you may wish to encourage young athletes to try cheaper options such as diluted juice, dried fruit (with water) or honey (with water).

Meal replacements

This category includes mainstream "fortified nutrition supplements" (such as Ensure) as well as sports-targeted products (such as EAS Myoplex and Met-Rx). They come either as powders designed to be mixed with water or milk, or as long-life ready-to-drink shakes in cartons.

Meal replacement drinks are essentially milk proteins (usually whey protein and/or casein), and maltodextrin and/or sugars, with added vitamins and minerals. Sports brands may also contain other ingredients, such as creatine and amino acids that claim to boost performance.

The main advantage of meal replacements is the fact that they supply fairly large amounts of energy, protein, vitamins and minerals in a convenient form. This makes them useful as post-training drinks or between-meal drinks. They can be prepared in advance and taken in a sports bag, then consumed after training or during break times at school. But regard them as supplemental to meals, rather than replacers of meals – the product name is a little misleading. Those who struggle to consume enough food to keep up their weight or to gain weight, may also want to consider adding these products to their daily food intake.

Check the ingredients on the label carefully as some products may contain substances such as creatine, which are not suitable for children and adolescents (*see* the section on creatine, above).

The main downside is their high cost, particularly those products targeted at the sports market. Mainstream "fortified nutrition supplements" are significantly cheaper and offer similar nutritional benefits, so may be a more realistic option for young athletes.

In conclusion, meal replacements are a safe and convenient way of getting extra energy and nutrients into the diet, particularly for those athletes who have high nutritional requirements.

Vitamin and mineral supplements

Young athletes' needs for vitamins and minerals are greater than those of non-active children. So it is tempting to think that supplements will enhance their health and performance.

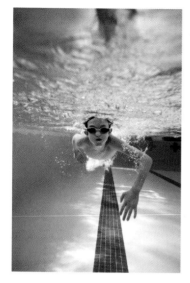

In fact, there is little scientific evidence to suggest that supplements benefit performance. The American College of Sports Medicine (ACSM) states that vitamin and mineral supplements are not needed if adequate energy to maintain body weight is consumed from a variety of foods (Rodriquez *et al.*, 2009). The consensus reports from the International Olympic Committee (IOC, 2004) and International Amateur Athletic Federation (IAAF, 2007) also conclude that most athletes are well able to meet their needs from food rather than supplements.

The ACSM concedes that supplementation may be warranted in athletes eating a restricted diet or an unbalanced diet that excludes one or more food groups. Some young athletes may fall into this category, in which case supplements could help make up any shortfall in their diet and improve their overall nutritional intake. In the short term, supplements would help improve their health, resistance to infection, and recovery.

Multivitamin and mineral supplements that provide about 100 percent of the recommended daily amounts (RDAs) are OK to take for insurance but could also be a waste of time if the athlete is consuming a healthy diet.

Young athletes should be guided to consume a varied and balanced diet, based on the "fitness food pyramid" described on page 35 in Chapter 1. They need to recognize the value of eating a variety of foods that includes whole grains, fruit, vegetables, dairy products and protein-rich foods. For individual advice on nutrition, consult a qualified nutritionist or dietitian (*see* the "References" section at the end of this chapter).

In conclusion, while multivitamin and mineral supplements are generally safe for children and adolescents when taken in the doses recommended for them, they shouldn't take the place of a healthy diet and certainly can't erase the effects of an unhealthy lifestyle.

Protein supplements

Protein supplements include protein powders, ready-to-drink protein shakes, and protein bars. These products provide a concentrated source of protein and may be based on milk proteins (whey or casein) or soy, or a mixture of these. All three types of protein contain high levels of essential amino acids, which are used to build body proteins.

It is important for young athletes to consume plenty of protein but it is better that they get it from food. Experts say they can get all they need from a balanced and varied diet. They need a little more protein than their non-athletic peers – around 1.2 to 1.4 g per 1 kg body weight (Boisseau *et al.*, 2007), that's 72–84 g for someone weighing 60 kg (*see* Chapter 1, page 17, "Protein"), which can be obtained from many foods. Consuming two or three portions of protein-rich foods daily – chicken, turkey, fish, meat, eggs, lean meat, cheese, milk, yogurt, beans, lentils and nuts – should provide enough protein. They will also get some protein from bread, pasta and breakfast cereals, which means, in practice, it is relatively easy for them to meet their daily requirement.

Protein supplements are generally considered safe but they will not necessarily build bigger and stronger muscles. This can be achieved only by combining a nutritionally adequate diet (that meets their protein needs) with a program of resistance training.

In conclusion, protein supplements are not necessary for young athletes, who should be encouraged to get their protein from a well-planned diet.

Sports Drinks

Sports drinks are designed to provide rapid fluid and fuel replenishment to the body during exercise. They contain between 4 and 8 g carbohydrate per 100 ml, plus electrolytes such as sodium and potassium. This concentration of carbohydrate is termed "isotonic" (which means the same concentration as body fluids) and is thought to be optimal for promoting the rapid absorption of water into the body (Coyle, 2004). Lower and higher concentrations both result in slower absorption rates.

The carbohydrate in sports drinks includes different combinations of sugars (such as glucose, sucrose and glucose syrup) and maltodextrin (complex carbohydrates derived from corn starch). These not only speed the absorption of fluid but also provide fuel for the muscles during exercise. The purpose of sodium in sports drinks is to stimulate drinking (salt makes us thirsty) and help the body retain the fluid better.

Many studies have shown that consuming sports drinks (instead of water) during exercise lasting more than an hour can help improve performance (e.g. Coyle, 2004), maintain blood glucose levels, provide fuel for the muscles, and reduce the risk of dehydration and hyponatraemia (low blood sodium levels) (Rodriquez *et al.*, 2009).

Research from the University of Texas found that drinking water during one hour of cycling improved performance by 6 percent compared with no water, but drinking a sports drink resulted in a 12 percent improvement on performance (Below *et al.*, 1995).

Young athletes should avoid sports drinks with caffeine, as these may result in side-effects (*see* page 48).

While sports drinks appear to be beneficial during prolonged exercise, their cost may be prohibitive for many young athletes. Similar benefits can be gained from less expensive alternatives, as in the examples that follow.

- Try mixing fruit juice with equal quantities of water. This produces an isotonic drink with around 6 g sugar per 100 ml. Add a pinch (0.5–1 g, one-eighth of a teaspoon) of ordinary salt if the young athlete sweats heavily.
- Dilute 200 ml squash with 800 ml water and 0.5–1 g (one-eighth of a teaspoon) salt (optional).
- Dissolve 40 g sugar and 0.5–1 g (one-eighth of a teaspoon) salt in 1 liter warm water. Add a little lemon or sugarfree juice for flavor.

Energy drinks

Energy drinks with caffeine are popular with adolescents, including athletes, who consume them before and during exercise in the belief that the drinks will give them a boost of energy, keep them alert and enhance their physical performance.

Energy drinks are essentially soft drinks with high levels of sugar and various combinations of caffeine, guarana, taurine, B vitamins and various herbs. They differ from sports drinks in that they include caffeine as well as carbohydrate. The sugar concentration is higher than that of sports drinks, around 10–12 g per 100 g, or 25–31 g per 250 ml can, but about the same concentration as most soft drinks (e.g. cola). This is too concentrated for the body to absorb quickly, which is why energy drinks cannot be considered sports drinks. They stay in the stomach longer than plain water or sports drinks, and so do not provide an efficient way of rehydrating the body. The US National Federation of State High School Associations advises young athletes to avoid energy drinks before, during and after exercise because of the potential risk of dehydration associated with them (NFHS, 2008).

Energy drinks contain about 80 mg caffeine per 250 ml, which is equivalent to a cup of coffee. However, some drinks come in larger cans, which means they may provide twice this amount of caffeine. Up to 85 mg daily is generally considered safe for children (*see* the section on caffeine, above) but higher doses are associated with side-effects: nervousness, an upset stomach, difficulty sleeping, anxiety, rapid heartbeat, dizziness and headaches. Since the effects of high levels of caffeine on children and adolescents participating in sports have not been studied, you should discourage young athletes from consuming energy drinks when exercising.

The bottom line is that energy drinks are not advisable for young athletes before, during or straight after exercise. They have not been shown to enhance exercise performance, and their high content of sugar and caffeine makes them unsuitable for proper hydration and delivery of carbohydrate. There is also little known about the added herbs and other substances in energy drinks.

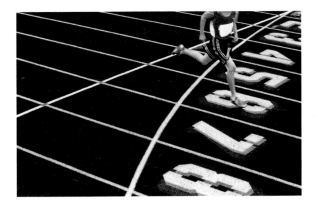

Omega-3 supplements

Omega-3s are essential fats found naturally in fish oils that play a vital role in healthy brain development and function, vision, learning ability, coordination and concentration. They are also important for regulating blood flow, blood pressure and the immune response, and protecting against cardiovascular disease. Recent research suggests that omega-3s may also help improve behavior in children with dyslexia, dyspraxia and ADHD.

Of interest to athletes, omega-3s increase the delivery of oxygen to muscles, and may help improve aerobic capacity and endurance, speed recovery and reduce joint stiffness. According to research at the University of California, supplementation with omega-3s for six weeks increases blood flow and oxygen delivery to the muscles during exercise (Walser *et al.*, 2006; Walser and Stebbins, 2008). In a study carried out at Western Washington University, people who consumed 4 g omega-3s per day for ten weeks while following a moderate exercise program increased their aerobic fitness by 11 percent, compared with controls who did not take supplements (Brilla and Landerholm, 1990).

The minimum requirement for omega-3s is 0.9 g a day, which you can get from one portion (140 g) of oily fish a week. The richest natural source of omega-3s is oily fish but research shows that many children are not eating the government's recommended levels – two portions of fish a week including one serving of oily fish such as mackerel, sardines, salmon, herring or fresh tuna. It is considered better that young athletes get their omega-3s from fish and other foods rather than taking supplements. Other food sources include nuts, seeds and green leafy vegetables (*see* Table 4.1). The omega-3s in plant foods are less potent than the omega-3s in fish but are still valuable to the body. The Vegetarian Society recommends vegetarians consume 4 g alpha linolenic acid (ALA) a day, equivalent to 50 g of walnuts or two teaspoons of flaxseed oil.

In conclusion, omega-3 fats are important for young athletes and they should be encouraged to get their daily quota from food sources. Omega-3 supplements are expensive but, for those who don't eat fish, they may be a convenient alternative.

Table 4.1 The omega-3 content of various foods

	g/100 g	Portion	g/portion
Salmon	2.5 g	100 g	2.5 g
Mackerel	2.8 g	160 g	4.5 g
Sardines (tinned)	2.0 g	100 g	2.0 g
Trout	1.3 g	230 g	2.9 g
Tuna (canned in oil, drained)	1.1 g	100 g	1.1 g
Cod liver oil	24 g	1 teaspoon (5 ml)	1.2 g
Flaxseed oil	57 g	1 tablespoon (14 g)	8.0 g
Flaxseeds (ground)	16 g	1 tablespoon (24 g)	3.8 g
Rapeseed oil	9.6 g	1 tablespoon (14 g)	1.3 g
Walnuts	7.5 g	1 tablespoon (28 g)	2.6 g
Walnut oil	11.5 g	1 tablespoon (14 g)	1.6 g
Pumpkin seeds	8.5 g	2 tablespoons (25 g)	2.1 g
Omega-3 eggs		1 egg	0.7 g
Typical kids' omega-3 supplement		2 capsules	0.3 g

References

Below, P.R. *et al.*, "Fluid and Carbohydrate Ingestion Independently Improve Performance During One Hour of Intense Exercise," *Med. Sci. Sports Ex.*, 27 (1995), pp. 200–210.

Boisseau, N. *et al.*, "Protein Requirements in Male Adolescent Soccer Players," *European Journal of Applied Physiology*, 100(1) (May, 2007), pp. 27–33.

Braun, H. *et al.*, "Dietary Supplement Use Among Elite Young German Athletes," *International Journal of Sport Nutrition and Exercise Metabolism*, 19(1) (2009), pp. 97–109.

Brilla, L.R. and Landerholm, T.E., "Effect of Fish Oil Supplementation and Exercise on Serum Lipids and Aerobic Fitness," *Journal of Sports Medicine and Physical Fitness*, 30(2) (June, 1990), pp. 173–180.

Coyle, E., "Fluid and Fuel Intake During Exercise," Journal of Sports Science, 22 (2004), pp. 39–55.

Food Standards Australia New Zealand (FSANZ), "Report from the Expert Working Group on the Safety Aspects of Dietary Caffeine" (2000), http://www.food-standards.gov.au/.

Heath and Welfare Canada, "Caffeine and Your Health" (2003), http://www.hc-sc.gc.ca/fn-an/securit/facts-faits/caffeine-eng.php.

International Association of Athletic Federations (IAAF) *Nutrition for Athletics: The 2007 IAAF Consensus Statement* (IAAF, 2007).

International Olympic Committee (IOC), "Proceedings of a Consensus Conference of the International Olympic Committee Medical Commission Nutrition and Sport Working Group (15–18 June, 2003), Lausanne, Switzerland," *Journal of Sports Science*, 22(1) (2004), pp. vii–x; 1–145.

Kreider, R.B., "Effects of Creatine Supplementation on Performance and Training Adaptations," *Mol. Cell. Biochem.*, 244 (2003), pp. 89–94.

Metzi, J.D. *et al.*, "Creatine Use Among Young Athletes," *Pediatrics*, 108(2) (2001), pp. 421–425.

National Federation of State High School Associations (NFHS), *Position Statement and Recommendations for the Use of Energy Drinks by Young Athletes* (NFHS, 2008).

Nieper, A., "Nutritional Supplement Practices in UK Junior National Track and Field Athletes," British Journal of Sports Medicine, 39(9) (2005), pp. 645–649.

Rodriquez, N.R., Di Marco, N.M. and Langley, S., "American College of Sports Medicine Position Stand: Nutrition and Athletic Performance. American Dietetic Association; Dietitians of Canada; American College of Sports Medicine," *Med Sci Sports Ex.*, 41(3) (2009), pp. 709–731.

Schänzer, W., *Analysis of Non-Hormonal Nutritional Supplements for Anabolic-Androgenic Steroids – an International Study*, Institute of Biochemistry, German Sport University Cologne (2002), http://multimedia.olympic.org/pdf/en_report_324.pdf.

Thomas, D.E. *et al.*, "Carbohydrate Feeding Before Exercise: Effect of Glycaemic Index," *International Journal of Sports Medicine*, 12 (2002), pp. 180–186.

Unnithan, V.B. *et al.*, "Is There a Physiologic Basis for Creatine Use in Children and Adolescents?," *J. Strength Cond. Res.*, 15(4) (2001), pp. 524–8.

Volek, J.S. and Kraemer, W.J., "Creatine Supplementation: Its Effects on Human Muscular Performance and Body Composition," *J. Strength Cond. Res.*, 10(3) (1996), pp. 200–210.

Walser, B. and Stebbins, C.L., "Omega-3 Fatty Acid Supplementation Enhances Stroke Volume and Cardiac Output During Dynamic Exercise," *European Journal of Applied Physiology*, 104(3) (2008), pp. 455–461.

Walser, B., Giordano, R.M. and Stebbins, C.L., "Supplementation with Omega-3 Polyunsaturated Fatty Acids Augments Brachial Artery Dilation and Blood Flow During Forearm Contraction," *European Journal of Applied Physiology*, 97(3) (2006), pp. 347–354.

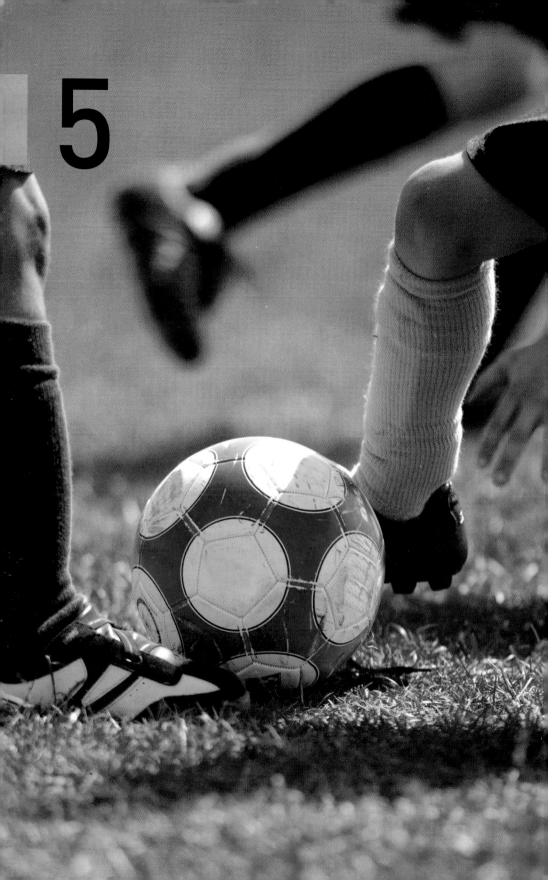

5

EATING FOR COMPETITION

Competitions are an integral part of most sports. They provide a reason for young athletes to train, goals to aim for, and opportunities for them to put into practice the fitness and the skills they have developed after weeks and months of hard training.

Whether they are competing in a race, a match, or a tournament involving several events, young athletes need to be well prepared nutritionally. What they eat and drink in the days and hours before a competition, as well as during the competition, can make a big difference to their performance. If they arrive at the event properly fueled and well hydrated, then they will have a competitive edge. But if they compete low on fuel and dehydrated, they will not put in their best performance. Planning ahead will help them have a successful competition and avoid food-related problems on the day. This chapter provides a nutrition guide to help young athletes prepare for competition.

The week before

During the last few days before a competition, young athletes should continue eating their normal diet. Make sure they stick to healthy eating principles as closely as possible during this time and that they stay well hydrated. They should focus on carbohydrate-rich foods in their diet – potatoes, pasta, rice and bread – to replenish glycogen levels after each training session, and drink plenty of water throughout the day. Encourage them to eat to their appetite – if they feel hungry, then provide bigger portions and healthy snacks, but do not "force feed" them if they are not hungry.

There is no need to manipulate the energy or carbohydrate content of their diet. Young athletes do not need to carbohydrate-load (consume extra carbohydrates in the last few days before a competition) – this is appropriate only for experienced athletes competing in endurance events lasting longer than 90 minutes.

For bigger competitions, they should, if possible, taper their training for a few days. This may mean reducing their training time and resting for a day or two before the event. The idea is to give the muscles an opportunity to fully repair themselves, and to refuel after an intense training period.

For smaller competitions, most coaches do not consider a taper necessary, apart from perhaps easing the training intensity of the last session. If young athletes are expected to compete frequently, say once a week, then it may be considered disruptive to their training schedule to taper for each competition. However, individual judgment would dictate whether and when the young athlete takes a rest day.

Q: SHOULD YOUNG ATHLETES CARBOHYDRATE LOAD BEFORE COMPETITIONS?

A: Carbohydrate loading is a nutrition and training strategy designed to maximize muscle glycogen stores before endurance competitions. Originally devised in the 1960s, it used to involve a three-day depletion phase (hard training combined with a low carbohydrate intake) followed by a three-day loading phase (light training combined with a high carbohydrate intake). Nowadays, experts advise omitting the depletion phase, as this provides no benefit. Carbohydrate loading has been shown to improve endurance performance by 2–3 percent in events lasting longer than 90 minutes, such as cycling, marathon running, longer-distance triathlon, cross-country skiing and long-distance swimming. But studies have been carried out only with adult men, not women, children or adolescent athletes, so it is not possible to say whether carbohydrate loading would work with young athletes. Given that few young athletes would be competing continually at a moderate or high intensity for longer than 90 minutes, carbohydrate loading is probably not a realistic option. For most sports, young athletes should aim to consume their usual diet prior to competition, perhaps increasing carbohydrate-rich foods and cutting down on high-fat foods during the last few days to facilitate glycogen storage.

Top tips for the week before a competition

- Stick to familiar foods and drinks – young athletes should not try anything new in the last few days in case it does not agree with them.
- Eat little and often – dividing their food into several small meals and snacks will make it easier to digest, keep their blood sugar levels steady and encourage muscle glycogen storage in preparation for the event.
- See that they don't skip meals – leaving long gaps between eating may result in low fuel stores before the competition.
- Ensure that they drink plenty of water – they need to keep well hydrated by drinking at least 1.5 liters a day, plus another 0.5 liters for each hour of exercise (they may need more in hot weather). Water is one of the healthiest options, but fruit juice and milk also count.
- They should avoid overeating late in the evening – big meals before bedtime may make them feel uncomfortable and lethargic the next day.
- Choose slow-burn meals – eating carbohydrate with protein provides sustained energy for all-day fueling. Suitable options include baked potato with beans, pasta with chicken, rice with fish.
- They should cut down on "empty calories" – reducing their intake of foods high in saturated fats and added sugars, such as candy, pastries, chips and fast foods, and instead eat nutrient-rich foods such as whole grains, fruit and vegetables which will prepare young athletes better for competition.

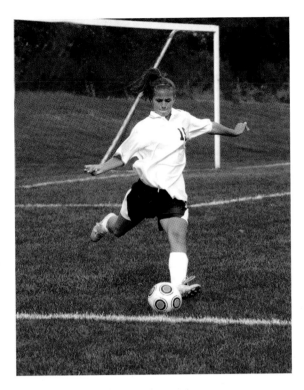

Test in training what they plan to do during the competition

Now is the time to rehearse their competition-day eating and drinking strategy. Whatever they plan to eat and drink during the competition should be rehearsed in training. They may experiment with different foods and drinks to find the types and amounts that suit them best. It's a good idea to research the foods and drinks to be provided at the venue so that you can plan what to take with you. Generally, it's safer to take your own supplies.

Eating on the move

Sometimes young athletes have to travel long distances to competitions, and spend hours in a car, bus, train or airplane. It's easy to forget to drink, and get dehydrated, so organize a traveling nutrition strategy.

Make sure they take their own supplies of food and drink for the journey. Do not rely on being able to find the right foods at stores en route or at the venue – healthy choices are often limited at these places.

If they're traveling abroad, it's important to avoid common food-poisoning culprits – chicken, seafood and meat dishes – unless you're sure they have been properly cooked and heated to a high temperature. As a rule of thumb, avoid anything that is lukewarm. Also, peel fruit and vegetables, stick to bottled water and avoid ice in drinks.

Q: SHOULD YOUNG ATHLETES EAT ANYTHING BEFORE AN EARLY-MORNING START ON COMPETITION DAY?

A: Many young athletes don't feel like eating, and struggle to eat a pre-competition meal early in the morning, partly due to nerves, partly due to the early start. But it's crucial that they consume at least a small amount of carbohydrate to raise blood glucose levels and top up muscle glycogen stores following the overnight fast. Competing on empty may result in low blood glucose levels, light-headedness, nausea and a poor performance. If a meal is out of the question, they should try to have a nutritious snack, such as wholewheat toast with honey, a granola bar or a banana. Alternatively, try a nutritious drink, such as milk, hot chocolate, flavored milk, a smoothie or a milkshake. Diluted juice or a sports drink would also be a suitable option, but steer them away from sweets, sugary drinks and energy drinks, which may have an unpredictable effect on their blood glucose level. Encourage them to drink water or diluted juice upon waking, and then to continue drinking little and often before competing.

Suitable foods for eating on the move include:

- sandwiches filled with peanut butter, banana, honey, chicken, tuna or cheese (keep in an insulated cooler bag if possible);
- rice cakes, oatcakes and wholewheat crackers;
- individual cheese portions;
- small bags of nuts – peanuts, cashews, almonds;

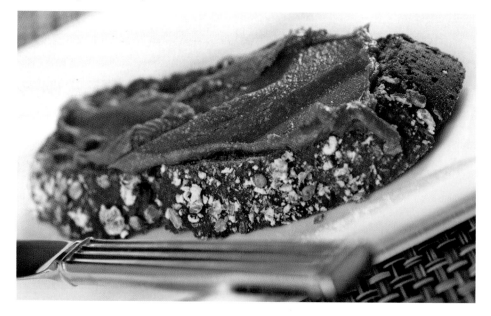

- fresh fruit – apples, bananas, grapes;
- dried fruit – apricots, raisins, mangoes;
- granola bars;
- prepared vegetable crudités, e.g. tomatoes, carrots (keep in a cooler bag if possible).

Suitable drinks on the move include:

- bottles of water;
- cartons of fruit juice;
- yogurt drinks;
- low-fat milk.

SUITABLE RESTAURANT MEALS AND FAST FOODS WHEN TRAVELING TO A COMPETITION

- Simple pasta dishes with tomato sauce
- Plain rice with vegetables, chicken or fish
- Pizza with tomato and vegetable toppings
- Simple noodle dishes (not fried)
- Baked potatoes with beans, tuna or cheese

RESTAURANT MEALS AND FAST FOODS TO AVOID

- Anything deep-fried
- Burgers and chips
- Chicken nuggets
- Pasta with creamy or oily sauces
- Battered fish and chips
- Hot dogs
- Fried chicken meals

> ## Q: ARE CAFFEINE-CONTAINING ENERGY DRINKS SUITABLE FOR YOUNG ATHLETES DURING COMPETITION?
>
> A: Many young athletes use caffeine-containing energy drinks before and during competition, in the belief that these drinks will give them a performance advantage. However, a 2009 review of health claims by the European Food Safety Authority (EFSA) dismissed the performance-enhancing claims made for these drinks: there is no evidence that they delay fatigue or enhance performance. Moreover, caffeine is not recommended for children and adolescents – studies have not yet demonstrated that it is safe or effective before or during exercise. It may have unpredictable side-effects, such as trembling, rapid heartbeat, dizziness, and headaches (see the section on caffeine in Chapter 4, page 87). The bottom line is that young athletes should steer away from caffeine-containing energy drinks as the side-effects may outweigh the potential benefits of caffeine for performance.

The day before

On the day before competition, the focus should be on topping up glycogen stores and ensuring that they are properly hydrated. In practice, this means avoiding strenuous exercise or training that may deplete their muscle fuel stores, although light exercise may be appropriate; eating carbohydrate-rich foods at each mealtime, with a nutritious snack in between, and drinking plenty of water. Below is a checklist to help them prepare for the next day.

Top tips for the day before competition
- Eat little and often – encourage them to eat several small meals throughout the day to maximize glycogen storage.
- Avoid fatty foods – fat-rich foods and fried foods, such as burgers, pies, nuggets and fries, take longer to digest and may overburden their digestive system, making them feel sluggish the next day.
- Don't try any new foods – make sure they play it safe by sticking to familiar and plain foods; they cannot risk an upset stomach. If traveling or eating out, steer them away from anything spicy or salty, or any meat or fish that may be undercooked.
- Hydrate – they should keep a water bottle handy so they remember to drink regularly throughout the day. This is especially important if they are traveling to the competition venue on this day, as it's easy to forget to drink. Their urine should be pale in color (see the "pee chart" presented in Figure 2.1) – if not, then they need to step up their fluid intake.
- Beware of the gas – it may be wise to avoid gas-producing foods (or combinations of foods) such as beans, lentils, cruciferous vegetables (broccoli, Brussels sprouts

and cauliflower), bran cereals and spicy foods the night before the competition. They may make them feel uncomfortable the next day.

- Don't over-indulge – too much food can play havoc with the digestive system and keep them awake at night. They should keep supper light, otherwise they risk feeling heavy and sluggish the next day.
- Get organized – don't rely on finding the right foods at stores en route nor at the venue. It's best that the young athletes take their own supplies for the journey as well for race day. They should also take extra water in case of delays.

Competition day

What they eat and drink on the day of the competition can make a big difference to young athletes' performance. If they have followed the nutrition rules presented above over the last few days, they should arrive at the competition fully fueled and well hydrated. But don't let them think it no longer matters what they eat, and that it's OK to indulge in sugary snacks. Too much sugar could play havoc with their blood glucose levels and result in flagging energy, fatigue and poor performance. For best performance, it's crucial that they continue paying attention to their food and drink intake before and during competition.

Eating before competing will help top up muscle glycogen stores and keep blood glucose levels steady during the competition. It is also important to replace fluids lost overnight.

Encourage them to have either a pre-competition meal or snack, depending on the start time. For early-morning starts, a normal-sized meal may not be feasible. Instead, they should eat a carbohydrate-rich meal the night before and then a healthy carbo-hydrate-rich snack (see the box entitled "Pre-competition snacks") about an hour before competing. This strategy will ensure they have enough fuel for the event.

If competitors feel nervous, encourage them to consume at least a small amount of food or a liquid meal (see the box entitled "How to cope with pre-competition nerves"), otherwise they risk low blood glucose levels while competing, light-head-edness and a poor performance.

Top tips for competition day

- They should eat 2–4 hours before competing – eating a carbohydrate-rich pre-event meal means that they will start exercise fully fueled.
- Steer them away from anything fried or high in fat, such as sausages, bacon, crois-sants and pastries. These foods take longer to digest (especially for competitors feeling nervous) and may sit heavy in their stomach, making them feel uncom-fortable during the competition. Try oatmeal, toast, cereal, milk, fruit or yogurt.

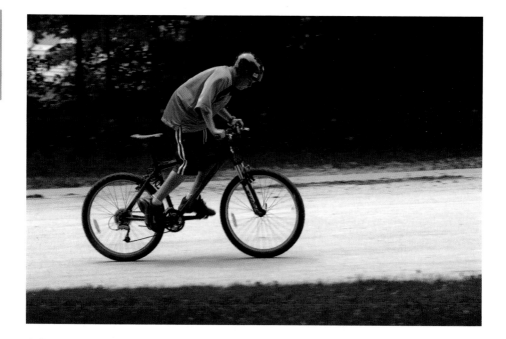

HOW TO COPE WITH PRE-COMPETITION NERVES

It's very common for young athletes to get pre-competition "nerves," which can dampen their appetite and make them feel nauseous. If they find it difficult to eat food during this time, try:

- liquid meals such as flavored milk, sports drinks, milkshakes, yogurt drinks and fruit smoothies;
- smooth, semi-liquid foods such as puréed fruit, yogurt, oatmeal, custard and rice pudding;
- bland foods such as oatmeal or rice cakes.

- Drink plenty – encourage them to have a drink upon waking. If possible, they should aim to drink 400–600 ml of water or diluted fruit juice (equal amounts of juice and water) during the two-hour period before the competition. This will allow sufficient time for the fluid to get absorbed and any excess to be excreted. As a hydration check, the urine should be pale in color before competing (see Figure 2.1).

- Plan an eating strategy – if they will be competing later in the day, or in several heats or matches, help them plan when to eat. Schedule meals and snacks around competition times; aim to leave two to four hours after a meal before competing, or about an hour after consuming a snack. Discourage skipping meals or constant grazing on sugary snacks otherwise their blood glucose may dip just before competing.

Q: WILL SWEETS AND CANDY HELP GIVE YOUNG ATHLETES EXTRA ENERGY WHEN COMPETING?

A: It's very common to see young athletes grazing on candy before competitions and during tournaments. Some are even encouraged to do so by well-meaning coaches and parents. However, the belief that these foods provide quick energy and benefit performance is unfounded. Eating too much sugar can cause big fluctuations in blood sugar levels and can, ironically, result in fatigue. Sugary foods and drinks produce a rapid rise in blood sugar levels, which in turn triggers the release of insulin to remove sugar from the bloodstream. Too much insulin can result in low blood sugar levels, light-headedness, nausea and early fatigue during exercise. Rather than giving them extra energy, sugar may sap their energy! If they need an energy boost while competing, opt for high-carbohydrate foods with a lower glycemic index, such as bananas, dried fruit and granola bars, that won't play havoc with their blood sugar levels. Grazing on sugary foods and drinks also increases the risk of tooth decay and acid erosion (dissolving) of the tooth enamel.

PRE-COMPETITION BREAKFASTS

- Oatmeal with dried fruit and honey
- Cereal with milk and yogurt
- Scrambled egg on toast
- Toast with honey, plus yogurt or a milky drink

PRE-COMPETITION SNACKS

- Dried fruit, e.g. raisins, apricots
- Granola bar
- Smoothie made with fruit and yogurt
- Yogurt
- Milkshake or milky drink
- Banana

Q: HOW CAN I MAKE SURE PLAYERS DRINK ENOUGH DURING LONG MATCHES?

A: Playing for longer than an hour can result in significant losses of fluid, which increases the risk of dehydration, early fatigue and a drop in performance. Avoid this by encouraging the players to start the match well hydrated (the "pee test" is a good way for them to self-monitor their hydration, *see* Figure 2.1) and to drink during breaks. Help them plan a drinking strategy – drink little and often during and immediately after the warm-up and during breaks in play. They should keep a water bottle handy, close to the field or playing area, somewhere within easy reach. If possible, they should take regular sips (or gulps), ideally every 15–20 minutes, depending on the sport, but without interrupting play! They should plan to start drinking as early as possible in the game and not wait until they feel thirsty before they start drinking.

Tournaments and multiple events

Many sporting competitions involve multiple games or a series of heats and finals on the same day or over consecutive days. To compete at their best, young athletes have to be prepared for different scenarios, and should have a flexible eating and drinking strategy, as the number of heats or games to be played may not be known, as this often depends on the outcome of individual heats and games. To further complicate matters, the exact start time of the event may change; or matches could go on for a shorter or longer duration than expected.

Whatever happens, it is important that they make recovery a priority. If they will be competing in more than one heat or game, they will have to refuel and rehydrate during the rest periods. These may vary in length and may not correspond to their usual mealtimes! Therefore, help them plan their food and drink consumption in advance, and make sure they have suitable drinks and foods ready. The key is to be organized and prepared. You should not rely on the food provided at the venue – healthy food and drink options may be limited or may be in short supply. Remember the rule: *do not try anything new on competition day.*

Encourage them to begin rehydrating and refueling as soon as possible after competing – the body restores glycogen faster during the 30 minutes after exercise, so the sooner they begin eating, the sooner the recovery process can take place. Fluids are needed for rehydration, while carbohydrates are needed for re-stocking muscle glycogen stores.

Rehydrating between events

It's crucial to replace fluids lost during competition as soon as possible. Failure to rehydrate between competitions can quickly lead to dehydration and result in fatigue and poor performance in the later heats or rounds. Encourage young athletes to follow the tips below for maintaining hydration.

- Drink around 250 ml within 30 minutes of completing the event
- Drink frequent small amounts rather than gulping a lot in one go – this promotes better retention of fluids
- If you pass only small volumes of dark-colored urine, increase your fluid intake – diluted juice or sports drinks will rehydrate faster than plain water

Suitable drinks for competition
- Water
- Fruit juice diluted half and half with water
- Sports drinks
- Milk
- Flavored milk

Fueling between events

If breaks between events are not long enough for a meal to be digested, plan for them to eat a light snack. Suitable options include sandwiches, wraps, light pasta dishes, fruit, rice cakes, dried fruit and mini-pancakes. These will be digested more easily and help maintain blood glucose levels. "Grazing" on lots of small nutritious snacks may be a better strategy if they have only short breaks between events. This may not satisfy their appetite as well as their usual meal plan, though, so, to avoid being hungry, they should try to have a small meal or a larger snack at a strategic time, such as during the longest break. Make sure they steer clear of slower-to-digest fatty foods such as burgers, fries, chips and cakes. Ideally, they should allow one to two hours between eating and competing.

COMPETITION-DAY STRATEGY FOR YOUNG ATHLETES

Do:
- stick to familiar foods and drinks;
- take your own foods and drinks wherever possible;
- have your normal meal two to four hours before competing – enough time to digest the food and for the stomach to feel comfortable;
- if too nervous to eat, try nutritious drinks, such as milk, fruit juice, smoothies, yogurt drinks and flavored milk, or light snacks;
- drink plenty of water or diluted juice before and after the event;
- always have drink bottles handy for regular fluid consumption.

Don't:
- skip meals – they may become light-headed or nauseous during the event and will not perform at their best;
- eat or drink anything new;
- have carbonated drinks – opt for non-carbonated drinks;
- eat high-fat foods like chips and hotdogs before the event;
- load up with sweets and sugary drinks all day!

Light meals for short breaks during competition
- Pasta – mix with a little pesto or tomato sauce; add any combination of peppers, tomatoes, cucumber, corn, nuts, tuna, chicken
- Sandwiches, wraps, rolls, pita bread; fill with a little chicken, tuna, cheese, salad or peanut butter

Refueling snacks during competition
- Bananas, melon, grapes, apples, pears
- Dried fruit, e.g. raisins, apricots, mango
- Rice cakes or crackers
- Mini-pancakes
- Granola bars, fruit bars
- Yogurt and yogurt drinks
- Small bags of nuts, e.g. peanuts, cashews, almonds

Practical considerations for competition day
- If competitors struggle to eat solid food due to nerves or excitement, encourage them to have nutritious drinks, such as milk, milkshake, smoothies or flavored milk.
- Ensure they practice their competition eating strategies in training so that they can be confident of avoiding stomach upsets on the day.

- The safest option is to take your own supplies. But you need to consider food freshness and perishability. Some foods, such as yogurts, milkshakes and cold meats, may be able to be kept cold for a few hours but should be consumed early in the day. Pack in an insulated bag or with a small ice pack if possible. Fragile food such as sandwiches and bananas should be packed in a protective container – soggy sandwiches and squashed bananas are not very appetizing! Non-perishable and "dry" food, such as rice cakes, granola bars and dried fruit, are usually the safest options for competitions.

Overnight recovery

If they will be competing the next day, or if they have finished their last competition, resist the temptation to celebrate the day's performance by indulging in treats or having a feast. Instead, use this overnight period as an opportunity for recovery. They should begin rehydrating and refueling as soon as possible after their competition finishes. The goal is to replenish fluid losses, restore muscle glycogen levels and repair damaged muscle tissue.

The first priority is to drink – rehydration takes place in the first 30–60 minutes following competition. Encourage them to drink water, diluted fruit juice, or, if they are dehydrated, sports drinks. The sodium in sports drinks will encourage better retention of fluid. Alternatively, eating salty foods such as sandwiches, toast or breakfast cereal along with water will promote fluid retention. Aim for 250–500 ml during this period and encourage drinking smaller volumes frequently rather than drinking a large volume in one go. If they are passing pale-colored urine, then this indicates that they are hydrated. But if they do not pass urine for two hours after competing, or only pass a small volume of dark-colored urine, this suggests that they are dehydrated. In this case, encourage drinking a sports drink or diluted fruit juice with a pinch of salt added (*see* page 53).

For major competitions, it may be feasible to get young athletes to weigh themselves before and after competing to estimate their fluid losses. Each 0.5 kg of weight loss is equivalent to 500 ml of fluid. They should replace this fluid gradually by drinking 750 ml for every 0.5 kg (1500 ml for every 1 kg) of weight lost.

To kick-start muscle glycogen reloading, encourage young athletes to have a healthy carbohydrate-rich snack as soon as possible after competing. This can include a small amount of protein as well as carbohydrate – combining protein and carbohydrate reduces the time it takes to recover and allows them to begin the next competition better prepared. The ideal recovery meal or snack should contain carbohydrate and protein in a 4:1 ratio. Good choices include low-fat milk, flavored milk, fruit with yogurt, a granola bar with a yogurt drink or a home-made milkshake.

Ideally, the recovery snack should be followed by a recovery meal within two hours but if this isn't possible, encourage them to have further frequent snacks until they resume their normal meal pattern. In fact, they should continue eating carbohydrate-rich snacks or meals until bedtime.

Suitable post-competition snacks
- 500 ml flavored milk
- 1 banana plus 500 ml of milk
- 2 pots (2 x 150 g) of fruit yogurt
- 1 granola bar plus 500 ml semi-skimmed milk
- A smoothie – blend 150 g yogurt, 1 banana and 150 ml fruit juice in a blender
- A cheese sandwich (2 slices bread, 40 g cheese)
- 60 g raisins and 50 g nuts
- 4 rice cakes with 20 g peanut butter plus 200 ml orange juice

Suitable post-competition meals
- Plain pasta dish with tomato pasta sauce, cheese (or chicken or fish) and vegetables
- Baked potato with tuna (or beans, cheese or chicken) and vegetables or salad
- Plain-cooked chicken with vegetables and rice
- Sandwiches, pita bread or wraps filled with cheese, meat or fish and salad
- Vegetable soup with cheese and bread
- Plain cooked fish, rice and salad
- Rice or noodles with vegetables and meat (or tofu or nuts)
- Omelet with potatoes and salad

Menu for ... a competition
The day before

Breakfast
A large bowl (80 g) wholegrain cereal with 300 ml milk and a banana

Snack
2 granola bars
A serving (about 100 g) of fresh fruit

Lunch
A wholewheat sandwich with 1 tablespoon (20 g) peanut butter and tomatoes
A pot (150 g) of fruit yogurt

Snack
3 rice cakes with 3 heaped teaspoons (30 g) honey, jam or chocolate spread
A serving (about 100 g) of fresh fruit
A yogurt drink (100 ml)

Supper
Pasta (85 g uncooked weight) with tomato sauce (100 g) and 2 tablespoons (40 g) grated cheese
Vegetables
Rice pudding (170 g, ready bought or home-made, *see* recipe page 139) with 100 g fresh or canned fruit

Snack
2 slices of wholewheat toast with margarine (20 g) and 1 tablespoon (20 g) honey or jam

Nutrition
2650 kcal
87 g protein
72 g fat (27 g saturates)
441 g carbohydrate

Competition day
Pre-competition breakfast (2–4 hours before the competition)
Oatmeal made with 85 g oats, 300 ml skimmed milk, 2 tablespoons (40 g) raisins, and 1 tablespoon (20 g) honey or sugar

During the competition (if appropriate)
500 ml fruit juice mixed with 500 ml water

Snacks between heats (if appropriate)
80 g dried fruit
4 rice cakes
3 granola bars

Immediately after competition
300 ml flavored milk or low-fat milkshake
2 bananas
A pancake (80 g, bought or home-made, *see* recipe for honey pancakes, page 142)

Post-competition meal (2 hours after)
Pasta (85 g uncooked weight) mixed with a little tomato sauce or pesto, chopped tomato/peppers/cucumber, and 85 g tuna or nuts
A serving (about 100 g) of fresh fruit

Nutrition
2726 kcal
84 g protein
49 g fat (10 g saturates)
520 g carbohydrate

MAIN MEALS

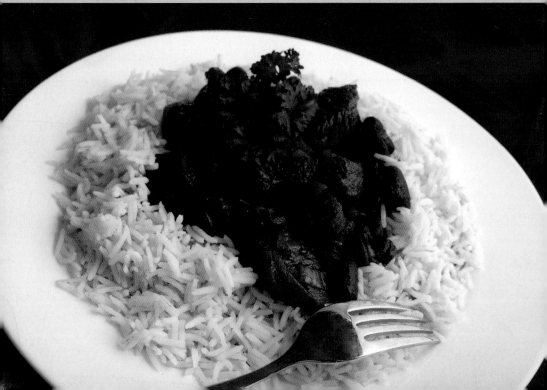

Turkey stir-fry with noodles

Makes 4 servings

300 g noodles
1 tablespoon olive oil
400 g turkey breast, cut into strips
2 green onions, trimmed, washed and diagonally sliced
2 garlic cloves, chopped
1 large carrot, cut into matchstick strips
200 g green cabbage, sliced into 2 cm pieces
Juice of 1 lime

1 Bring a large pot of water to the boil, add the noodles and cook according to instructions. Drain and transfer to a bowl.
2 Rub a little oil around a wok or large non-stick frying pan, then place over high heat. Add the turkey strips and stir-fry for 8–10 minutes until golden and thoroughly cooked. Transfer to a plate, cover and keep warm.
3 Reheat the pan. When hot, add the remaining ingredients, except the turkey, noodles and lime juice. Stir-fry for 2 minutes until the cabbage has wilted. Return the turkey and noodles to the pan and stir in the lime juice.
4 Serve immediately.

Nutrition (per serving)
433 kcal
33 g protein
8.3 g fat (<1 g saturates)
60 g carbohydrate

Chicken salad pita with yogurt dressing

Makes 4 servings

4 boneless skinless chicken breasts
300 g low-fat yogurt
Salt and freshly ground pepper
1 teaspoon ground cumin
Juice of ½ lemon
2 garlic cloves, crushed
2 teaspoons liquid honey
4 wholewheat pita breads
75–100 g mixed salad greens
100 g cucumber, chopped
½ red pepper, deseeded and sliced
Handful fresh coriander leaves

1 Cut each chicken breast into 4–5 slices. Measure 100 g of the yogurt into a bowl. Season and add a little of the cumin. Add the chicken, coat well, cover and marinate for 1–2 hours if possible.
2 Heat a grill or saucepan to medium–high and grill or sauté the chicken, turning halfway through, for about 8 minutes, or until cooked through and golden. Leave to cool a little. Meanwhile, mix the remaining yogurt and cumin, the lemon juice, garlic and honey, and season.
3 Halve and split the pitas, and fill with some of the salad greens and cucumber. Divide the chicken between the pitas, spoon the dressing over, and garnish with the pepper and coriander. Serve with any extra salad on the side.

Nutrition (per serving)
389 kcal
43 g protein
3.9 g fat (1.1 g saturates)
49 g carbohydrate

Tomato and tuna pasta

Makes 4 servings

225 g can tuna in olive oil
1 onion, finely sliced
1 garlic clove, chopped
1 red or yellow pepper, chopped
2 x 400 g cans chopped tomatoes
2 tablespoons tomato purée
300 g penne pasta
2 tablespoons basil leaves, roughly torn
20 g Parmesan

1 Drain the oil from the tuna into a medium pan and put the tuna to one side.
2 Heat 1 tablespoon of the oil and fry the onion on low heat for about 10 minutes, until softened. Add the garlic and cook for 1 minute. Add the peppers and canned tomatoes, and stir everything together. Simmer over medium heat for 15 minutes to reduce the sauce.
3 Meanwhile, bring a large pot of lightly salted water to the boil and cook the pasta according to instructions. Drain and toss with the sauce. Garnish with basil and Parmesan shavings, if using, to serve.

Nutrition (per serving)
458 kcal
26 g protein
13 g fat (2.7 g saturates)
63 g carbohydrate

Chili con carne

Makes 4 servings

1 tablespoon olive oil
2 onions, chopped
1 garlic clove, chopped
2 carrots, peeled and grated
2 sticks celery, chopped
450 g lean ground beef
½ teaspoon chili powder
A little dried oregano
3 tablespoons tomato purée
410 g can red kidney beans
400 ml water

1 Heat the olive oil in a large saucepan, add the onions, garlic, carrots, celery and beef, and cook for about 5 minutes until the beef has browned and the onion softened. Add the chili powder and oregano, and cook for another 1–2 minutes.
2 Add the tomato purée, beans and water, cover and cook over low heat for about 1 hour. Serve the chili with cooked rice.

Nutrition (per serving)
250 kcal
19 g protein
11 g fat (3.2 g saturates)
19 g carbohydrate

Chicken casserole

Makes 4 servings

1 tablespoon olive oil
2 onions, roughly chopped
1 garlic clove, crushed
2 x 400 g cans chopped tomatoes
125 g button mushrooms
3 zucchini, sliced
A handful of fresh basil
8 chicken thighs

1 Preheat oven to 200°C. Heat the oil in a frying pan, add the onions and cook for 2 minutes, then add the garlic and 50 ml water, and simmer for 3–4 minutes until soft.
2 Place the onion mixture into a casserole dish with the tomatoes, mushrooms and zucchini, then scatter with the basil leaves. Add the chicken thighs and turn to coat in the tomato mixture. Bake for 40–45 minutes, until the chicken is thoroughly cooked through and the juices run clear. Serve with cooked rice or boiled new potatoes.

Nutrition (per serving)
237 kcal
28 g protein
12 g fat (2.8 g saturates)
6.0 g carbohydrate

Rice with chicken and green beans

Makes 4 servings

400 g can condensed cream of chicken soup
150 g long-grain rice, rinsed
500 g boneless skinless chicken breasts, cut into bite-sized pieces
250 g frozen green beans
1 tablespoon chopped fresh chives

1 Empy the soup into a wide, deep frying pan, fill the can with water and rinse out into the pan. Stir in the rice and chicken, and bring to the boil. Simmer, uncovered, for 15–17 minutes, stirring occasionally, until the sauce has reduced and the rice and chicken are just cooked.
2 Meanwhile, cook the frozen beans according to instructions. Fold into the chicken and rice with the chives, and season with salt and freshly ground black pepper.

Nutrition (per serving)
377 kcal
41 g protein
8.0 g fat (1.7 g saturates)
37 g carbohydrate

Tuna pasta salad

Makes 4 servings

300 g pasta
4 ripe tomatoes, roughly chopped
175 g frozen peas
1 tablespoon olive oil
2 handfuls of baby spinach leaves
1 teaspoon balsamic vinegar
210 g can tuna in water, drained
Small handful basil leaves, roughly torn

1 Cook the pasta in a large pan of boiling water, according to instructions.
2 Meanwhile in a small pan combine the tomatoes, peas and olive oil. Heat gently for 5 minutes.
3 Stir the baby spinach leaves and balsamic vinegar into the tomato mixture.
4 Drain the pasta and return to the pan, then add the vegetables, tuna and basil. Stir to combine and serve.

Nutrition (per serving)
373 kcal
23 g protein
5.0 g fat (<1 g saturates)
64 g carbohydrate

Chicken with chickpeas and tomatoes

Makes 4 servings

1 tablespoon olive oil
1 onion, chopped
2 carrots, thickly sliced
2 boneless, skinless chicken breasts, cut into strips (about 300 g)
400 g can chopped tomatoes
300 ml hot chicken stock
410 g can chickpeas, drained and rinsed
Handful of fresh coriander, chopped

1 Heat the olive oil in a large, heavy-based pan, and add the onion and carrots. Cover the pan and sweat the vegetables over a low heat for 10 minutes. Remove the vegetables from the pan and set them to one side. Increase the heat slightly, add the chicken strips and cook for a few minutes until golden brown.
2 Add the vegetables back to the pan, then add the tomatoes and the stock. Stir in the chickpeas, season and bring to a simmer for 20 minutes, covered, until the chicken is cooked through. Stir in the coriander, and serve with baked potatoes or crusty bread.

Nutrition (per serving)
237 kcal
29 g protein
7.4 g fat (1.3 g saturates)
15 g carbohydrate

Pasta and shrimp

Makes 4 servings

350 g dried tagliatelle pasta
3 tablespoons olive oil
3 garlic cloves, thinly sliced
350 g raw shelled tiger shrimp
Zest and juice of ½ lemon
2 tablespoons tomato purée
4 tablespoons freshly chopped parsley
2 tablespoons freshly grated Parmesan

1　Cook pasta in a large pot of boiling water according to instructions.
2　Meanwhile, heat half the oil in a large frying pan or wok. Fry the garlic slices for 1–2 minutes, add the shrimp and cook, stirring, for 2–3 minutes until they turn pink.
3　Drain the cooked pasta and add remaining olive oil, lemon zest and juice, tomato purée, parsley and shrimp. Season and toss to mix. Serve immediately, sprinkled with freshly grated Parmesan.

Nutrition (per serving)
476 kcal
29 g protein
12 g fat (2.5 g saturates)
68 g carbohydrate

Quick tuna and vegetable pasta

Makes 4 servings

1 tablespoon olive oil
1 onion, sliced
300 g pasta
300 g broccoli, chopped
210 g can tuna, drained

1　Heat the olive oil in a pan. Add the onion and cook over medium heat for 8–10 minutes until golden and soft.
2　Meanwhile, cook the pasta in a large pan of boiling water according to instructions. Add the chopped broccoli to the pasta for the last 5 minutes of cooking. Drain, then return to the pan.
3　Add the tuna to the pasta with the onions and toss everything together before serving immediately.

Nutrition (per serving)
353 kcal
22 g protein
5.0 g fat (<1 g saturates)
58 g carbohydrate

Chicken and vegetable stir-fry

Makes 4 servings

1 large onion
2 large carrots
150 g baby corn
150 g sugarsnap peas
4 skinless boneless chicken breasts
2 tablespoons vegetable oil
1 teaspoon curry powder
120 ml chicken stock or water
2 tablespoons tomato ketchup

1   Peel, halve and thinly slice the onion. Peel and cut the carrots in half lengthwise then cut into thin slices. Halve the baby corn and sugarsnap peas.
2   Cut the chicken breasts into thin strips.
3   Heat a wok or frying pan over high heat and add the oil. Add the chicken and curry powder and stir-fry for 2–3 minutes, until the chicken is cooked through.
4   Add the onion and carrot and stir-fry for 2 minutes more. Then add the corn and sugarsnap peas and stir-fry for a further 2 minutes.
5   Add the stock and tomato ketchup and simmer for 1–2 minutes. Serve at once with cooked rice or noodles.

Nutrition (per serving)
286 kcal
40 g protein
10 g fat (2.0 g saturates)
9.4 g carbohydrate

Lamb stew

Makes 4 servings

1 tablespoon olive oil
800 g lean lamb, cut into 5 cm (2 in) pieces
1 onion, finely diced
2 carrots, finely diced
4 celery sticks, finely diced
2 leeks, thinly sliced
2 tablespoons flour
Freshly ground black pepper
1 tablespoon Worcestershire sauce
800 g potatoes unpeeled

1   Heat the olive oil in a large saucepan. Add the lamb and cook until it is brown all over. Then transfer it to a plate.
2   Reduce the heat. Add the vegetables and sauté them for 10 minutes, stirring frequently.
3   Remove from heat, add the meat, sprinkle in the flour and mix it up thoroughly. Pour in enough hot water to cover the meat and vegetables, stir well and return to the heat.
4   Preheat the oven to 100°C
5   Bring the meat and vegetables to a boil, stirring often as the gravy thickens. Season and add the Worcestershire sauce. Then remove it from the heat. Transfer to an oven-proof casserole dish.
6   Thinly slice the potatoes, either by hand or with a mandolin. Layer them carefully to completely cover the meat and vegetables.
7   Place the stew in the oven and cook for 2 hours. The potatoes should be golden on top and the gravy bubbling up nicely around the sides.

Nutrition (per serving)
487 kcal
30 g protein
21 g fat (8.5 g saturates)
48 g carbohydrate

Chicken balti

Makes 4 servings

75 g red lentils
1 tablespoon of olive oil
2 carrots
1 mango, peeled, stoned and cubed
2 tomatoes, chopped
½ teaspoon of chili powder
1 teaspoon of ground coriander
450 g chicken breast, boned, skinned and cubed
2 tablespoons of fresh coriander, chopped

1 Place the lentils in a saucepan and add enough water to barely cover them. Bring to the boil and then simmer for about 10 minutes, until they are soft but not mushy. Drain well and set aside.
2 Heat the oil in a large non-stick frying pan. Add the carrots and cook over a medium heat for 4–5 minutes.
3 Add the mango, tomatoes, chili powder, ground coriander and chicken. Cook for 8–10 minutes, stirring occasionally.
4 Add the cooked lentils and cook for a further 2 minutes, or until the chicken is cooked through.
5 Garnish with fresh coriander before serving with plain basmati rice or naan bread.

Nutrition (per serving)
294 kcal
39 g protein
6.8 g fat (1.6 g saturates)
21 g carbohydrate

Fish pie

Makes 4 servings

450 g boned white fish
Milk
500 g potatoes
400 g sweet potatoes
25 g butter or margarine
225 g corn
125 g frozen peas
1 tablespoon parsley, chopped

For the cheese sauce:
25 g butter or margarine
25 g flour
600 ml semi-skimmed milk
125 g Cheddar cheese
A little salt, freshly ground black pepper
½ teaspoon Dijon mustard

1 Preheat the oven to 200°C.
2 Poach the fish in just enough milk to cover, for about 5 minutes. Drain and then roughly flake the fish.
3 Peel the potatoes and sweet potatoes and cut into large chunks. Boil until tender, drain, then mash with the butter or margarine and, if necessary, a little milk until smooth.
4 Meanwhile cook the corn (if frozen) and peas in a saucepan for about 3–4 minutes, then drain and place in a deep dish along with the fish.
5 Make the cheese sauce by melting the butter or margarine in a saucepan. Stir in the flour then gradually add the milk, whisking continuously over a low heat until the sauce has thickened. Stir in most of the cheese, salt, pepper and mustard.
6 Pour the sauce over the fish and vegetable mixture, and top with the mashed potato. Sprinkle with the remaining cheese. Bake for 20 minutes or until golden brown.

Nutrition (per serving)
664 kcal
38 g protein
27 g fat (15 g saturates)
73 g carbohydrate

VEGETARIAN MAIN MEALS

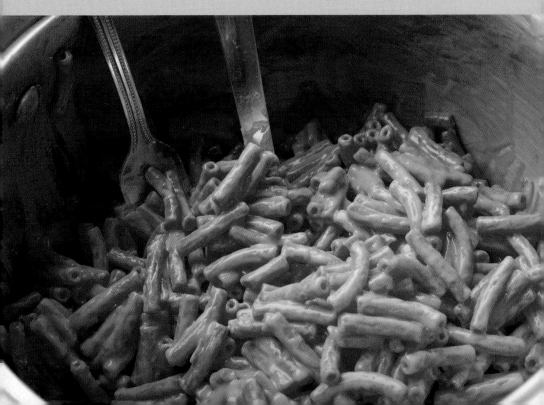

Pizza

Makes 1 pizza

For the pizza base:
225 g white flour
½ packet active dry yeast
½ teaspoon salt
175 ml warm water
1 tablespoon olive oil

For the tomato sauce:
1 tablespoon olive oil
1 small onion, finely chopped
1 garlic clove, crushed
1 tin (400 g) chopped tomatoes
1 tablespoon tomato purée
1 teaspoon dried basil
½ teaspoon sugar
Pinch of salt and freshly ground black pepper
125 g mozzarella, sliced or grated Cheddar cheese

Suggested toppings: sliced tomatoes, halved cherry tomatoes, sliced red or yellow peppers, sliced mushrooms, corn, sliced onion, olives, sliced zucchini, baby spinach leaves, spring onion

1 If making the dough by hand, prepare the yeast accoding to instructions and set aside. Mix the flour and salt in a large bowl. Make a well in the center and add the oil, yeast and half the water. Stir with a wooden spoon, gradually adding more liquid until you have a pliable dough. Turn the dough out onto a floured surface and knead for about 5 minutes until you have a smooth and elastic dough. Place the dough in a clean, lightly oiled bowl, cover with a tea towel and leave in a warm place for about 1 hour or until doubled in size.
2 If you are using a bread machine, put the ingredients in the machine and follow the instructions supplied.
3 Turn out the dough; knead briefly before rolling out on a floured surface to the desired shape. Transfer to an oiled pizza pan or baking tray and finish shaping by hand. The dough should be approx. 5 mm thick. Let the dough rise for 30 minutes.
4 Meanwhile, make the tomato sauce. Heat the oil and sauté the onion and garlic for 5 minutes. Add the chopped tomatoes, tomato purée, basil, sugar, salt and pepper. Continue to simmer for 5–10 minutes or until the sauce has thickened a little. Spread the sauce on the pizza base. Sprinkle with the cheese and any additional toppings from the list above.
5 Bake at 200°C for 15–20 minutes until the cheese is bubbling and golden brown.

Nutrition (per ¼ pizza)
341 kcal
14 g protein
13 g fat (5.0 g saturates)
46 g carbohydrate

FOR A QUICK MEAL, TRY ANY OF THE FOLLOWING ALTERNATIVE PIZZA BASES

- Ready-made pizza base
- An English muffin, toasted and split horizontally
- Focaccia bread, halved horizontally and toasted
- Ciabatta loaf, halved horizontally and toasted
- Wholewheat or white pita bread, split horizontally and lightly toasted
- French bread, sliced in half horizontally and toasted

Macaroni and cheese

Makes 4 servings

300 g macaroni
125 g frozen peas
25 g flour
300 ml milk (whole or semi-skimmed)
½ teaspoon Dijon mustard
85 g aged Cheddar, grated
Freshly ground black pepper

1 Preheat the oven to 200°C.
2 Cook the macaroni in boiling water according to instructions, adding the frozen peas during the last 3 minutes of cooking time. Drain.
3 Blend the flour with a little of the milk in a small bowl. Gradually add the remainder of the milk.
4 Heat the milk and flour mixture in a saucepan, stirring continuously until the sauce just reaches the boil and has thickened.
5 Remove from the heat, stir in the mustard, half the cheese and freshly ground pepper to taste.
6 Stir in the macaroni and peas. Spoon into an ovenproof dish, Sprinkle with the remaining cheese and bake for 15–20 minutes until the top is bubbling and golden.

Nutrition (per serving)
426 kcal
19 g protein
10 g fat (5.7 g saturates)
69 g carbohydrate

Ratatouille with butternut squash

Makes 4 servings

2 onions, cut into wedges
500 g zucchini, sliced
2 peppers (1 red, 1 yellow), cut into wide strips
1 small butternut squash (about 300 g), peeled, seeded and cut into wedges
250 g tomatoes, quartered
2–3 garlic cloves, chopped
Few sprigs fresh thyme, roughly chopped
4 tablespoons olive oil
Freshly ground black pepper
Grated Cheddar cheese

1 Preheat the oven to 200°C.
2 Place the vegetables, tomatoes, garlic and thyme in a large, deep roasting pan. Drizzle with the olive oil and turn gently so that they are evenly coated. Roast in the oven for about 40 minutes or until the vegetables are beginning to soften and turn golden brown. Stir occasionally as they cook.
3 When the vegetables are ready, remove from the oven and season with freshly ground black pepper. Sprinkle with a little grated cheese. Serve with baked potatoes.

Nutrition (per serving)
159 kcal
3.5 g protein
12 g fat (1.8 g saturates)
10 g carbohydrate

Pasta, broccoli and cheese casserole

Makes 4 servings

300 g pasta
375 g broccoli
2 level tablespoons flour
600 ml semi-skimmed milk
½ teaspoon Dijon mustard
Freshly ground black pepper
85 g aged Cheddar cheese, grated

1 Preheat the oven to 180°C. Cook the pasta according to instructions.
2 Cut the broccoli into small florets and boil until tender (about 5 minutes). Drain.
3 Blend the flour with a little of the milk in a small bowl. Gradually add the remainder of the milk, stirring to ensure a smooth sauce. Pour into a saucepan and heat, stirring constantly until the sauce just reaches the boil and has thickened.
4 Remove from the heat, stir in the mustard and freshly ground black pepper to taste.
5 Stir in the drained pasta and broccoli. Pour into a large ovenproof dish and sprinkle with the cheese. Place in the oven and bake for 20–25 minutes, until golden brown and bubbling.

Nutrition (per serving)
495 kcal
24 g protein
15 g fat (7.0 g saturates)
71 g carbohydrate

Pasta with chickpeas and spinach

Makes 4 servings

500 g pasta
235 g bag baby spinach
410 g can chickpeas, drained and rinsed
350 g jar pasta sauce
Freshly ground black pepper
125 g cheese, grated

1 Bring a large pot of water to a boil. Add the pasta and cook according to instructions. Remove from the heat and drain thoroughly. Stir in the spinach and allow to wilt.
2 Place the chickpeas in a medium pan with the tomato sauce. Gently bring to a boil over low heat. Turn off the heat.
3 Tip the pasta into a serving dish and pour the hot pasta sauce and chickpea mixture over the top, then toss together and season with black pepper. Top each serving with grated cheese.

Nutrition (per serving)
572 kcal
28 g protein
14 g fat (5.1 g saturates)
88 g carbohydrate

Vegetarian stir-fry

Makes 4 servings

2 tablespoons light soy sauce
2 tablespoons wine vinegar
1 tablespoon sugar
1 garlic clove, crushed
350 g tofu, cut into chunks
250 g Thai fragrant rice
1 tablespoon oil
1 onion, sliced
1 red and 1 yellow pepper, seeded and sliced
200 g broccoli, cut into florets
1 heaped teaspoon flour
4 tablespoons cold water
1–2 teaspoons toasted sesame seeds

1   Mix the soy sauce, vinegar, sugar and garlic, and then add the tofu and coat well. Cover and marinate for 1–2 hours if possible.
2   When ready to cook, drain the tofu, reserving the marinade. Put the rice to cook, according to packet instructions.
3   Heat a wok with half the oil over a high heat. Add the tofu (you might need to do this in batches). Stir-fry for 1–2 minutes until golden then remove to a warm plate. Add the remaining oil to the pan, then the onions, peppers and broccoli. Stir-fry for 3 minutes or until just tender.
4   Stir the flour and water into the reserved marinade and add to the wok, along with the tofu. Cook briefly until thickened. Add a little hot water if needed to give a rich sauce. Serve with the rice, sprinkled with sesame seeds.

Nutrition (per serving)
404 kcal
15 g protein
9.0 g fat (1.2 g saturates)
70 g carbohydrate

Three-bean pasta

Makes 4 servings

2 tablespoons oil
1 onion, finely chopped
1 celery stalk, finely chopped
1 parsnip, chopped
1 garlic clove, crushed
1 bay leaf
400 g can mixed beans, drained
400 g can chopped tomatoes
1 tablespoon tomato purée
2 tablespoons roughly chopped herbs, such as basil, thyme, rosemary
450 ml vegetable stock
300 g small pasta
25 g Parmesan, freshly grated, to serve

1   Heat the oil in a saucepan and add the onion, celery, parsnip and garlic. Add a splash of water and cover. Cook over a low to medium heat for 5–10 minutes until the vegetables are soft and translucent.
2   Add the bay leaf, beans, chopped tomatoes, tomato purée, herbs and stock. Season, cover and bring to the boil. Simmer for 15 minutes.
3   Add the pasta to the pan and stir. Put the lid back on and bring to a simmer. Cook for 10 minutes.
4   Remove the bay leaf and stir half the Parmesan into the pan. Spoon into bowls and sprinkle with the remaining cheese.

Nutrition (per serving)
455 kcal
18 g protein
9.7 g fat (2.4 g saturates)
79 g carbohydrate

Pasta and tomato salad

Makes 4 servings

300 g pasta
2 tablespoons olive oil
4 sun-dried tomatoes in oil, drained
4–5 spring onions
225 g cherry tomatoes
8–12 basil leaves
8–12 black olives
125 g aged Cheddar cheese, cut into cubes

1 Cook the pasta in a large pot of boiling water until al dente, according to instructions. Drain the pasta, refresh under cold running water, then drain again and transfer to a large bowl. Stir in the olive oil to prevent the pasta from sticking.
2 Slice the sun-dried tomatoes. Trim and finely shred the spring onions. Halve the cherry tomatoes. Tear the basil leaves into pieces. Add to the pasta along with the olives and toss to mix.
3 Toss with the cubes of cheese and accompany with a leafy green salad

Nutrition (per serving)
378 kcal
9.9 g protein
13 g fat (1.9 g saturates)
59 g carbohydrate

Roast tomato pasta

Makes 4 servings

300 g pasta
500 g cherry tomatoes
2 tablespoons olive oil
Salt and freshly ground black pepper
60 g pine nuts
A large handful of basil leaves, torn
Freshly grated Parmesan cheese

1 Preheat the oven to 240°C.
2 Bring a large pot of water to a boil and cook the pasta according to instructions. Drain the pasta well.
3 Meanwhile, cut the tomatoes in half and arrange them in a large roasting pan, cut side up. Drizzle with olive oil. Season with salt and black pepper. Roast in the oven for 15 minutes until the tomatoes are softened and lightly caramelized. Meanwhile, put the pine nuts on a cookie sheet and roast for 5–7 minutes until lightly golden.
4 Mix the pasta with the tomatoes, basil and pine nuts, then stir in a little extra oil if the pasta needs it. Serve sprinkled with a generous amount of Parmesan.

Nutrition (per serving)
478 kcal
16 g protein
21 g fat (3.8 g saturates)
61 g carbohydrate

Pasta with mushrooms

Makes 4 servings

350 g pasta
1 tablespoon olive oil
1 onion, sliced
200 g button mushrooms
3 tablespoons crème fraîche
2 tablespoons freshly chopped flat-leafed parsley

1   Cook the pasta in a large pot of boiling water, according to instructions.
2   Meanwhile, heat the olive oil in a pan. Add the sliced onions and fry gently for 3 minutes until starting to soften. Add the button mushrooms and fry for 5–6 minutes. Drain the pasta, return to the pot and add the onions and mushrooms.
3   Stir in the crème fraîche and parsley. Toss everything together, season to taste and heat through to serve.

Nutrition (per serving)
392 kcal
12 g protein
11 g fat (4.8 g saturates)
67 g carbohydrate

Pasta with butternut squash

Makes 4 servings

1 butternut squash, halved, peeled and roughly chopped
2 tablespoons olive oil
Zest of 1 lemon
Salt and freshly ground black pepper
350 g pasta
75 g Cheddar cheese, grated
Fresh basil leaves, torn

1   Preheat the oven to 200°C.
2   Place the butternut squash in a roasting pan, drizzle with olive oil and add the lemon zest. Sprinkle with a little salt and freshly ground black pepper. Cook in the oven for about 20 minutes, until soft and the edges just begin to color.
3   In a large pot of boiling water, cook the pasta according to instructions, drain and tip back into the pan with a little of the cooking water. Toss with the roasted squash, then stir through the cheese and more black pepper if needed. Sprinkle with fresh basil to serve.

Nutrition (per serving)
458 kcal
16 g protein
14 g fat (5.1 g saturates)
73 g carbohydrate

Pesto pasta with vegetables

Makes 4 servings

300 g pasta
50 g pine nuts
1 tablespoon olive oil
1 crushed garlic clove
250 g sliced mushrooms
2 sliced zucchini
250 g cherry tomatoes
3 tablespoons pesto
25 g Parmesan

1 Cook the pasta according to instructions.
2 Gently toast the pine nuts in a frying pan for a few minutes. Remove. Add olive oil to the pan, then the garlic, mushrooms and zucchini. Add a splash of water to the pan, then cover and cook for 4–5 minutes. Uncover and add cherry tomatoes, then cook for a further 1–2 minutes.
3 Drain the pasta and return to the pot. Add the vegetables and pine nuts, the pesto and Parmesan to the drained pasta. Toss well to combine, and serve immediately.

Nutrition (per serving)
527 kcal
20 g protein
25 g fat (5.0 g saturates)
61 g carbohydrate

Vegetable pasta casserole

Makes 4 servings

225 g pasta
2 large carrots, thinly sliced
175 g broccoli, cut into small florets
125 g canned corn
1 tablespoon olive oil
60 g Cheddar cheese, grated
1 tablespoon sunflower seeds, toasted
60 g fresh bread crumbs

For the cheese sauce:
1 level tablespoon flour
300 ml semi-skimmed milk
½ teaspoon Dijon mustard
60 g aged Cheddar cheese, grated
Freshly ground black pepper

1 Preheat oven to 200°C.
2 Cook the pasta according to instructions. Drain and transfer to an ovenproof dish.
3 Place the carrots in a pan of boiling water and cook for 3 minutes. Add the broccoli and cook until just tender. Drain well.
4 Make the cheese sauce. Blend the flour with a little of the milk in a small bowl. Gradually add the remainder of the milk, stirring to ensure a smooth sauce. Pour into a saucepan and heat, stirring constantly until the sauce just reaches the boil and has thickened.
5 Remove from the heat, stir in the mustard, cheese and freshly ground black pepper to taste. Stir the cooked vegetables, corn and cheese sauce into the pasta and season.
6 Mix the oil, cheese and sunflower seeds into the bread crumbs, then sprinkle on the vegetables. Cook in the oven for 20 minutes, until the topping is golden.

Nutrition (per serving)
537 kcal
21 g protein
19 g fat (8.2 g saturates)
76 g carbohydrate

Bean and vegetable stew

Makes 4 servings

1 tablespoon olive oil
225 g mushrooms
2 carrots, sliced
1 large potato, cubed
225 g green beans, chopped
1 teaspoon dried thyme
2 garlic cloves, crushed
700 ml vegetable stock
Seasoning
225 g frozen broad beans
410 g can Roman beans (or any other variety of beans)

1   Heat the oil in a large pan, add the mushrooms, carrots, potato and green beans, and gently fry for 3–4 minutes.
2   Add the thyme, garlic and vegetable stock. Bring to a boil, then simmer uncovered for 20 minutes until the vegetables are tender.
3   Stir in all the beans and then cook for a further 10 minutes. Serve with baked potatoes.

Nutrition (per serving)
224 kcal
12 g protein
6.8 g fat (1.0 g saturates)
31 g carbohydrate

Thai vegetable curry

Makes 4 servings

400 ml can reduced-fat coconut milk
2 tablespoons Thai green curry paste
2 carrots, sliced
300 g broccoli, divided into small florets
150 g sugarsnap peas, trimmed
150 g baby corn, cut in half
100 g unsalted cashew nuts

1   Pour the coconut milk into a wide pan, then stir in the green curry paste and bring to a simmer.
2   Add the carrots and simmer gently for 10 minutes.
3   Add the broccoli florets, peas and sliced baby corn, and simmer gently for a further 5 minutes.
4   Stir in the cashew nuts, and serve with boiled rice or rice noodles.

Nutrition (per serving)
243 kcal
11 g protein
15 g fat (2.8 g saturates)
17 g carbohydrate

Vegetable chili

Makes 4 servings

2 tablespoons oil
1 onion, sliced
2 red peppers, seeded and cut into chunks
1 tablespoon mild chili powder
1 large carrot, peeled and cut into chunks
2 medium potatoes, peeled and cut into
chunks
400 g can chopped tomatoes
200 ml hot vegetable stock
410 g can red kidney beans in chili or
tomato sauce
50 g green beans, trimmed and halved

1 Heat the oil in a large pan. Add the onion
   and cook on medium heat for 5 minutes
   until softened, then add the peppers and
   cook for 2 minutes. Add the chili powder
   and stir for 1 minute. Stir in the carrot and
   potatoes, then add the tomatoes and
   stock and simmer for 15–20 minutes.
2 Add the red kidney beans and simmer for
   a further 5 minutes. Finally, add the green
   beans and simmer for 5–10 minutes or
   until all the vegetables are tender. Serve
   with basmati rice.

Nutrition (per serving)
249 kcal
9.0 g protein
6.8 g fat (1.0 g saturates)
40 g carbohydrate

Vegetable risotto

Makes 4 servings

15 g butter
1 tablespoon olive oil
2 red peppers, sliced
300 g risotto rice
1 clove garlic, crushed and chopped
750 ml hot vegetable stock
200 g green beans
125 g spinach
50 g Parmesan shavings

1 Melt butter and oil in a pan, add the
   peppers, rice and garlic. Mix well. Add a
   ladleful of hot stock and stir well, simmer
   and repeat until all stock is added and the
   rice is just cooked.
2 Slice beans and add for the final 3 minutes
   of cooking. Stir in the spinach and serve
   topped with Parmesan.

Nutrition (per serving)
420 kcal
12 g protein
11 g fat (4.9 g saturates)
72 g carbohydrate

SOUP

Vegetable soup

Makes 4 servings

2 tablespoons olive oil
1 onion, chopped
1 garlic clove, crushed
1 liter vegetable stock
750 g vegetables, e.g. sliced carrots, diced
butternut squash, green beans, frozen peas,
broccoli florets, cauliflower florets
Salt and freshly ground black pepper
1 tablespoon fresh herbs, e.g. chives, parsley,
basil, thyme

1 Heat the olive oil in a large pot. Add the
   onion and garlic and cook for about
   5 minutes. Add the stock and the prepared
   vegetables, bring to the boil and then
   simmer for about 20 minutes or until the
   vegetables are soft.
2 Turn off the heat. Season and stir in the
   herbs.
3 For a smooth soup, purée in a blender or
   food processor, or using a hand blender.
   For a chunky, thick soup, purée half the
   soup and return to the pot.

Nutrition (per serving)
115 kcal
1.3 g protein
6.1 g fat (1.0 g saturates)
15 g carbohydrate

Butternut squash soup

Makes 4 servings

2 tablespoons olive oil
1 onion, chopped
1 medium (about 450 g) butternut squash,
peeled and chopped
1 large carrot, sliced
1 medium potato, peeled and chopped
900 ml vegetable stock
1 teaspoon (5 ml) grated fresh ginger (or
½ teaspoon ground ginger)
Freshly ground black pepper

1 Heat the oil and sauté the onion for about
   5 minutes, until transparent.
2 Add the butternut squash, carrot and
   potato, and cook for a further
   2–3 minutes.
3 Add the stock and ginger and bring to the
   boil. Turn down the heat and simmer for
   20 minutes or until the vegetables are
   tender.
4 Remove from the heat. Purée the soup
   using a hand blender or food processor.
5 Season with black pepper.

Nutrition (per serving)
143 kcal
2.5 g protein
5.9 g fat (<1 g saturates)
21 g carbohydrate

Carrot and coriander soup

Makes 4 servings

1 tablespoon (15 ml) extra virgin olive oil
1 onion, finely sliced
1 garlic clove, crushed
500 g carrots, sliced
700 ml vegetable stock
1 bay leaf
Salt and freshly ground black pepper
A handful of fresh coriander, roughly chopped

1   Heat the olive oil in a heavy-based saucepan over moderate heat. Add the onion and sauté gently for about 5 minutes until it is translucent.
2   Add the garlic and cook for a further 1–2 minutes. Add the carrots, stock and bay leaf to the pan, stir, then bring to a boil. Simmer for 15 minutes or until the vegetables are tender.
3   Allow the soup to cool slightly for a couple of minutes. Remove and discard the bay leaf. Purée the soup using a hand blender or conventional blender. Season to taste, then stir in the fresh coriander.

Nutrition (per serving)
93 kcal
<1 g protein
5.9 g fat (1 g saturates)
9.9 g carbohydrate

Pea soup

Makes 4 servings

1 tablespoon of butter
1 tablespoon olive oil
1 small onion, finely chopped
Salt and freshly ground pepper
600 ml vegetable stock
400 g fresh or frozen peas
A handful of mint leaves, roughly chopped
4 tablespoons low-fat plain yogurt, to serve

1   Melt the butter with the oil in a large saucepan over a medium heat. Add the onion, season, cover and cook very gently for 15 minutes or until completely soft.
2   Add the stock and bring to a gentle simmer, then add the peas and simmer for 10 minutes until they are soft. Remove from the heat, add the chopped mint, and purée.
3   Serve hot or chilled, garnished with a swirl of plain yogurt, a sprig of mint and lots of black pepper, accompanied by crusty wholewheat bread.

Nutrition (per serving)
141 kcal
7.6 g protein
7.1 g fat (2.8 g saturates)
12 g carbohydrate

Lentil soup

Makes 4 servings

2 tablespoons olive oil
1 large onion, chopped
1–2 garlic cloves, crushed
225 g red lentils
1 liter vegetable stock
Juice of 1 lemon
Salt and freshly ground black pepper

1 Heat the olive oil in a heavy-based saucepan over medium heat. Add the onion and garlic and cook for about 5 minutes until translucent.
2 Add the lentils and vegetable stock, and bring to a boil. Reduce the heat and simmer for 20 minutes. Add the lemon juice, bring back to a boil and simmer for a further 10 minutes until the lentils are soft.
3 Season to taste, ladle into bowls.

Nutrition (per serving)
228 kcal
13 g protein
6.2 g fat (<1 g saturates)
32 g carbohydrate

Tomato soup

Makes 4 servings

2 tablespoons olive oil
1 onion, chopped
1 large carrot, grated
1 red pepper, chopped
1 large potato, peeled and cubed
2 garlic cloves, crushed
1 can (400 g) chopped tomatoes
750 ml boiling water or hot vegetable stock
1 teaspoon (5 ml) sugar
Freshly ground black pepper

1 Heat the oil and sauté the onion for 2–3 minutes in a large saucepan. Add the carrot, red pepper, potato and garlic, and cook for a further 5 minutes.
2 Add the tomatoes, water and sugar. Simmer for about 20 minutes or until the vegetables are soft.
3 Purée the soup using a hand blender or food processor, and season with the black pepper.

Nutrition (per serving)
125 kcal
2.4 g protein
5.9 fat (<1 g saturates)
16 g carbohydrate

DESSERTS

Apple crumble

Makes 4 servings

700 g cooking apples
2 tablespoons fine sugar
2 tablespoons water
2 teaspoons ground cinnamon
100 g flour
50 g light brown sugar
50 g rolled oats
50 g butter or margarine

1 Preheat the oven to 190°C.
2 Peel, core and thinly slice the apples, and place in a 1-liter ovenproof casserole dish. Toss with the sugar. Pour over 2 tablespoons boiling water.
3 Place the cinnamon, flour, brown sugar and rolled oats in a mixing bowl. Add the butter or margarine and rub into the mixture until it resembles bread crumbs.
4 Sprinkle the topping over the apples and bake for 40–45 minutes until golden brown. Serve with a spoonful of vanilla ice cream.

Nutrition (per portion)
271 kcal
7.4 g protein
9.2 g fat (4.6 g saturates)
42 g carbohydrate

Apple pancakes

Makes 4 servings

100 g self-rising flour
2 eggs, beaten
150 ml milk
3 tablespoons fine sugar
Small amount of oil
25 g butter or margarine
2 eating apples, thinly sliced

1 Put the flour in a mixing bowl, make a well in the center, add the eggs and a little milk, and mix until smooth. Slowly add the rest of the milk and beat to a smooth batter. Stir in 1 tablespoon of the sugar.
2 Lightly oil a frying pan and heat. Drop a large tablespoonful of mixture onto the hot pan, cook for 2–3 minutes until golden brown underneath and almost set on top, turn over and cook other side until golden. Keep warm while making remaining pancakes.
3 Melt the butter or margarine in a small frying pan and fry the apple slices until golden. Add the remaining sugar and stir until dissolved. Serve with the pancakes.

Nutrition (per portion)
378 kcal
4.5 g protein
12 g fat (6.6 g saturates)
68 g carbohydrate

Baked bananas with apricots

Makes 4 servings

4 ripe bananas
125 g dried apricots
1 tablespoon honey
4 tablespoon toasted flaked almonds

1 Preheat the oven to 190°C. Cut four rectangles of foil, 25 x 30 cm each.
2 Peel the bananas. Cut a slit in the banana lengthwise, not quite cutting all the way through. Place each one on a piece of foil.
3 Put the apricots into a food processor. Add 4 tablespoons of water and the honey, and process for a few seconds to make a smooth purée.
4 Spoon the purée over the bananas and fold over the foil, twisting the ends to make sealed parcels. Arrange on a baking tray and bake for 10 minutes.
5 Carefully open the foil parcels and sprinkle with the almonds.
6 Serve with yogurt or ice cream.

Nutrition (per portion)
235 kcal
4.6 g protein
6.1 g fat (<1 g saturates)
43 g carbohydrate

Oats, banana and yogurt dessert pots

Makes 4 servings

6 tablespoons instant oats
2 tablespoons granulated sugar
2 ripe bananas
400 ml plain yogurt

1 Sprinkle the oats on a baking tray with the sugar. Toast gently for 3–4 minutes, turning frequently until golden and crisp.
2 Mash the bananas and mix with the yogurt. Layer into four dessert dishes with the toasted oats.

Nutrition (per portion)
203 kcal
7.3 g protein
2.5 g fat (<1 g saturates)
40 g carbohydrate

Plum clafoutis

Makes 4 servings

500 g plums
20 g butter
25 g flour
25 g fine sugar
3 eggs
350 ml semi-skimmed milk

1 Heat the oven to 180°C.
2 Halve the plums and remove the pits. Butter a shallow baking dish and add the plums.
3 In a blender, mix the flour, sugar, eggs and milk until smooth and creamy.
4 Pour over the plums and bake in the oven for 30–35 minutes.
5 Leave to cool a little and then dust lightly with sugar.

Nutrition (per portion)
235 kcal
10 g protein
11 g fat (5.0 g saturates)
27 g carbohydrate

Rice pudding

Makes 4 servings

50 g arborio or short-grained rice
600 ml milk (whole or semi-skimmed)
40 g granulated sugar
Grated nutmeg

1 Preheat the oven to 150°C.
2 Put the rice, milk and sugar in a 1.8-liter pie dish. Stir the mixture, then sprinkle with grated nutmeg.
3 Bake for 1½ hours, or until the milk has been absorbed and there is a light-brown skin on top of the pudding. Serve with spicy fruit compôte (*see* recipe, page 140) or canned apricots.

Nutrition (per portion)
154 kcal
5.9 g protein
2.7 fat (1.6 g saturates)
28 g carbohydrate

Baked apples

Makes 4 servings

4 cooking apples (e.g., Spy, McIntosh)
60 g raisins
6–8 dried apricots, chopped
1 tablespoon liquid honey
2 tablespoons pecans, chopped

1 Preheat the oven to 190°C.
2 Core the apples, and with a sharp knife, lightly score the skin around the middle, just enough to pierce the skin.
3 In a small bowl, combine the dried fruit, honey and pecans. Fill the cores of the apples, then place them in a baking dish. They should fit snugly side by side. Add 2 tablespoons of water, cover loosely with foil then bake for 45–60 minutes.
4 Check a few times during cooking, adding a little extra water if the dish becomes dry.
5 Serve warm with plain yogurt.

Nutrition (per portion)
284 kcal
4.3 g protein
9.3 g fat (<1 g saturates)
49 g carbohydrate

Spicy fruit compôte

Makes 4 servings

1 tablespoon liquid honey
1 teaspoon ground cinnamon
Juice of 1 lemon
500 g dried fruit, e.g. apricots, apples, pears, prunes, figs and cranberries, roughly chopped

1 Put the honey, cinnamon, lemon juice and 600 ml boiling water in a large pan. Bring to a boil and simmer for 5 minutes. Add the dried fruit and then simmer for a further 5 minutes. Remove from the heat and leave to steep until ready to serve.
2 Serve with yogurt or vanilla ice cream.

Nutrition (per portion)
226 kcal
5.0 g protein
<1 g fat (<1 g saturates)
53 g carbohydrate

BAKING

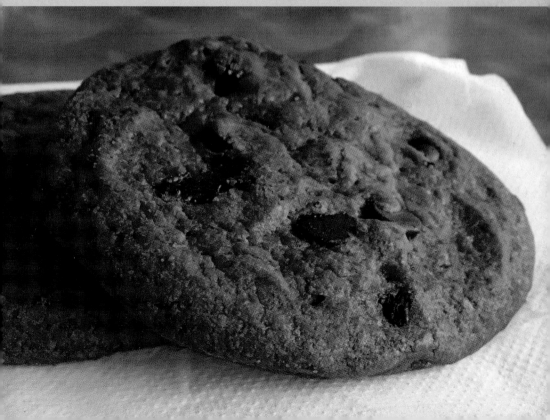

Honey oat squares

Makes 12 slices

200 g butter or margarine
200 g granulated sugar
200 g honey
400 g rolled oats
50 g raisins or candied cherries

1 Preheat the oven to 180°C. Grease a 20 x
   30 cm cake pan.
2 Put the butter, sugar and honey in a
   saucepan and heat, stirring occasionally,
   until the butter has melted and the sugar
   has dissolved. Add the rolled oats and
   raisins or cherries, and mix well.
3 Transfer the mixture to the prepared pan
   and spread to about 2 cm thick. Smooth
   the surface with the back of a spoon.
4 Bake in the oven for 15–20 minutes, until
   lightly golden around the edges but still
   slightly soft in the middle.
5 Let cool in the pan, then turn out and cut
   into squares.

Nutrition (per slice)
383 kcal
4.3 g protein
17 g fat (2.8 g saturates)
57 g carbohydrate

Banana and walnut loaf

Makes 10 slices or 12 muffins

2 medium ripe bananas
125 g butter
175 g dark brown sugar
2 eggs
1 teaspoon vanilla extract
1 teaspoon ground cinnamon
250 g flour
1 teaspoon baking powder
3 tablespoons milk
125 g walnuts

1 Preheat the oven to 180°C. Grease a loaf
   pan or use a large muffin pan.
2 Mash the bananas. Cream the butter and
   sugar until smooth and then beat in the
   mashed bananas. Add the eggs, vanilla
   and cinnamon, and mix well.
3 Add the flour, baking powder and milk,
   and mix until smooth. Fold in the walnuts.
4 Spoon the mixture into the pan and bake
   for about 50 minutes, until the loaf is
   crusty on the top and a skewer inserted
   into the middle comes out clean. Cool in
   the pan and then turn out on to a cooling
   rack. For muffins, cook for 20–25 minutes.

Nutrition (per slice)
370 kcal
6.0 g protein
21 g fat (7.7 g saturates)
43 g carbohydrate

Blueberry muffins

Makes 18 muffins

375 g flour
1 tablespoon baking powder
150 g fine sugar
2 large eggs
90 g melted butter
284 ml buttermilk
200 g blueberries

1 Preheat the oven to 200°C and line two
   muffin pans with paper liners.
2 Sift the flour and baking powder into a
   large bowl and stir in the sugar.
3 In another bowl, whisk together 2 large
   eggs, melted butter and buttermilk. Fold
   this mixture into the flour and stir the
   blueberries through. Spoon into muffin
   pan and bake for 20–25 minutes until
   cooked and golden.

Nutrition (per muffin)
152 kcal
2.8 g protein
5.1 g fat (2.9 g saturates)
25 g carbohydrate

Fruit buns

Makes 12 buns

500 g white bread flour
1 teaspoon salt
2 teaspoons pumpkin pie spice
100 g fine sugar
7 g packet active dry yeast
100 g dried mixed fruit
50 g butter
250 ml milk, plus 3 tablespoons milk
1 large egg, beaten

1 Prepare the yeast according to instructions
   and set aside. In a large bowl, sift together
   the flour, salt, spice and 50 g of the sugar
   and fruit. In a small pan, melt the butter,
   then add the milk and heat until tepid – it
   should just feel warm to the touch.
2 Make a well in the dry ingredients, stir in
   the milk, then the egg and yeast, and mix
   to form a soft dough. Tip the dough out on
   to a floured work surface and knead for
   5–8 minutes until smooth and elastic.
3 Divide into 12 equal pieces and shape
   each into a ball. Place a little way apart on
   an oiled baking sheet, use a knife to cut a
   cross in top of each. Cover with oiled
   plastic wrap and leave to rise in a warm
   place for about 1½ hours until doubled in
   size.
4 Preheat the oven to 190°C. Bake for
   20–25 minutes or until golden brown.
5 When the buns are nearly ready, heat the
   remaining sugar and milk with 3
   tablespoons water in a small pan, stirring
   until the sugar dissolves. Boil for 1 minute.
   Remove the buns from the oven and brush
   with the glaze. Leave to cool on a wire
   rack. Serve warm, spread with butter.

Nutrition (per bun)
246 kcal
6.4 g protein
4.9 g fat (2.6 g saturates)
47 g carbohydrate

Raspberry muffins

Makes 12 muffins

4 tablespoons sunflower oil
75 ml milk
1 large egg
150 g self-raising flour
100 g fine sugar
175 g fresh or frozen raspberries
4 tablespoons icing sugar, sifted
2 teaspoons lemon juice

1 Preheat the oven to 200°C. Line a six-muffin pan with paper liners.
2 Mix the oil, milk and egg together. Sift the flour and sugar into a bowl. Add the liquid and half the raspberries to the flour and briefly mix until just coming together. Spoon into the muffin liners and sprinkle the remaining raspberries over. Bake for 25–30 minutes.
3 Cool the muffins on a wire rack. Sift the icing sugar into a bowl, stir in lemon juice to make a runny icing. Drizzle the icing over the muffins and leave to set. Pack the muffins into an airtight container. They will keep for 2–3 days.

Nutrition (per muffin)
145 kcal
2.0 g protein
4.5 g fat (<1 g saturates)
26 g carbohydrate

Almond and apricot cake

Makes 12 slices

150 g margarine
150 g sugar
2 eggs
100 g ground almonds
175 g self-raising flour
300 ml plain low-fat yogurt
100 g dried apricots

1 Preheat the oven to 180°C. Line a 20 cm round cake pan with baking parchment paper.
2 Beat the margarine and sugar until pale and creamy.
3 Add the eggs, almonds, flour and yogurt, and combine well.
4 Roughly chop the apricots and then fold in to the mixture.
5 Spoon into the prepared pan and bake in the oven for 30–40 minutes or until a skewer inserted in to the center comes out clean. Leave to cook in the pan for 10 minutes, remove from the pan and cool on a wire rack.

Nutrition (per slice)
284 kcal
5.9 g protein
17 g fat (3.0 g saturates)
30 g carbohydrate

Date slices

Makes 12 slices

350 g pitted dates, roughly chopped
200 ml water
A piece of lemon rind
150 g butter or margarine
225 g wholewheat flour
125 g rolled oats
85 g brown sugar

1   Preheat the oven to 200°C. Grease a rectangular 28 x 18 cm pan.
2   Place the dates, water and lemon rind in a small saucepan, bring to a boil and simmer for 8–10 minutes, until very soft. Discard the lemon peel.
3   Rub the butter or margarine into the flour until the mixture resembles breadcrumbs. Stir in the oats and sugar.
4   Press half the crumble mixture into the prepared pan. Spread the dates over and then cover with the remaining crumble.
5   Bake in the preheated oven for 20–25 minutes or until lightly browned. Cut into 16 slices.

Nutrition (per slice)
255 kcal
4.2 g protein
12 g fat (6.6 g saturates)
36 g carbohydrate

Chocolate chip oatmeal cookies

Makes 20 cookies

125 g butter or margarine
85 g brown sugar
85 g granulated or fine sugar
1 egg
½ teaspoon vanilla essence
150 g flour
½ teaspoon baking powder
60 g rolled oats
100 g chocolate chips

1   Preheat the oven to 180°C and grease one or two baking sheets (or use baking parchment paper).
2   Cream together the butter or margarine and the sugars until light and smooth.
3   Beat in the egg and vanilla.
4   Sift together the flour and baking powder into a bowl. Add the rolled oats and fold into the liquid mixture, mixing well. Stir in the chocolate chips.
5   Place spoonfuls on to the baking sheets, about 2.5 cm apart, and bake for 8–10 minutes or until lightly browned. Allow to cool for about 5 minutes before gently lifting with a spatula onto a wire rack.

Nutrition (per cookie)
146 kcal
1.8 g protein
7.2 g fat (4.2 g saturates)
20 g carbohydrate

Fruit loaf

Makes 10 slices

300 ml/½ pint milk
175 g golden brown sugar
75 g raisins
250 g dried apricots or plums, chopped, or
use more raisins
3 tablespoons corn syrup
2 tablespoons liquid honey
350 g self-raising flour, sifted
1–2 tablespoons ground ginger or pumpkin
pie spice, sifted
3 tablespoons apricot jam

1 Preheat the oven to 180°C. In a large
   bowl, combine the milk and sugar, then
   mix in the fruit. Drizzle in the corn syrup
   and honey, and stir well. Next, add the
   flour and spice, and mix again until
   combined.
2 Spoon into a loaf pan and place in the
   oven for about 45 minutes to an hour,
   until golden brown and a skewer comes
   out clean when poked in the middle. Leave
   to cool in the pan for 10 minutes before
   turning out on to a wire rack. Melt a little
   apricot jam and brush it over the cake.
   Slice to serve.

Nutrition (per slice)
317 kcal
5.1 g protein
1.1 g fat (<1 g saturates)
76 g carbohydrate

Wholewheat bread

Makes 16 slices

500 g wholewheat bread flour
1 teaspoon salt
1 teaspoon active dry yeast
1 teaspoon sugar
1 tablespoon olive oil
325 ml warm water

1 Prepare the yeast according to the
   instructions, and set aside. In a large bowl,
   mix together the flour, salt and sugar. Add
   the oil, yeast and water, and roughly mix
   into the flour. Stir together until you have
   a soft dough.
2 Lightly flour your hands and the work
   surface. Transfer the dough onto the
   floured work surface and knead well for
   about 10 minutes until it feels smooth and
   pliable.
3 Leave the dough covered with a tea towel
   in an oiled bowl, in a draft-free place, for it
   to double in size (this should take about an
   hour).
4 Turn the dough out on to a floured surface
   and knead the dough firmly for several
   minutes.
5 Shape the dough and put it into an oiled
   loaf pan, or place it on a greased baking
   sheet.
6 Cover with a clean tea towel and leave the
   dough to rise for about 25 minutes in a
   warm place. Preheat the oven to 220°C.
7 Bake in a preheated oven for 35–40
   minutes. It should sound hollow when
   tapped on the base.

Nutrition (per slice)
103 kcal
4.0 g protein
1.4 g fat (<1 g saturates)
20 g carbohydrate

Focaccia

Makes 8 servings

500 g bread flour
1½ teaspoons active dry yeast
2 teaspoons sugar
1 teaspoon salt
2 tablespoons olive oil
315 ml lukewarm water
A few stems of rosemary
A few black olives
A little coarse sea salt

1   Prepare the yeast according to instructions, and set aside. Put the flour, sugar and salt in a large bowl. Add the yeast and 1 tablespoon of the olive oil and gradually mix in the water using a wooden spoon, then mix with your hands to make a soft dough.
2   Transfer to a floured surface and knead for 8–10 minutes, or until the dough is smooth and satiny.
3   Put the dough back into the bowl, cover with plastic wrap and set aside in a warm spot for 45–60 minutes until the dough has doubled in size.
4   Transfer the dough onto a floured work surface and knead once or twice until smooth. Divide into two pieces and pat each into a rough oval. Place on two large oiled baking sheets. Cover with a clean tea towel and set aside to rise for another 30 minutes.
5   Using your fingertips, dimple the surface of the dough, pushing in about halfway. Roughly cut the rosemary sprigs and press into the holes in the dough, along with the olives. Spoon the remaining olive oil over each piece of dough and sprinkle with the coarse salt.
6   Bake in the oven for 15 minutes until the focaccia are golden brown and sound hollow when tapped. Serve warm or cold.

Nutrition (per serving)
248 kcal
7.2 g protein
4.0 g fat (<1 g saturates)
49 g carbohydrate

Walnut bread

Makes 2 loaves/16 slices

350 g wholewheat bread flour
200 g white bread flour, plus extra for dusting
7 g active dry yeast
1½ teaspoons salt
1 teaspoon sugar
360 ml lukewarm water
1 tablespoon olive oil
150 g walnuts, coarsely chopped

1   Prepare the yeast according to instructions, and set aside. Mix the flours, salt and sugar in a large bowl. Stir in the water, yeast and olive oil. Gradually add up to 100 ml more water until the flour is incorporated and the dough is soft.
2   Turn out the dough on to a lightly floured surface and knead for 8–10 minutes, or until smooth and elastic. Shape into a ball.
3   Put the dough back in the bowl, cover with plastic wrap and leave in a warm place until doubled in size. Meanwhile, lightly dust a large baking tray with flour.
4   Punch down the dough, turn it out onto a floured surface and knead for 1 minute. Shape the dough into a rectangle and sprinkle with the walnuts. Knead for a few more minutes, or until the nuts are evenly distributed.
5   Cut the dough in half and form each into a ball. Transfer to the baking tray and flatten. Cover with a tea towel and leave to rise for 15 minutes. Preheat the oven to 220°C.
6   Bake for 10 minutes, reduce the temperature to 190°C, and bake for a further 25–35 minutes or until the bases sound hollow when tapped. Transfer to a wire rack and leave to cool.

Nutrition (per slice)
181 kcal
5.6 g protein
7.8 g fat (<1 g saturates)
24 g carbohydrate

USEFUL WEBSITES

http://www.momsteam.com/nutrition
This website for parents of young athletes has a section on nutrition.

http://www.powerbar.com/
This commercial website contains sound and useful articles on nutrition for adult and teen athletes.

http://kidshealth.org/
This US website offers expert food and fitness advice for parents, teenagers and kids.

http://www.nourishinteractive.com/
This website geared towards children is an educational site with games, challenges and puzzles that teach children about nutrition.

http://www.ayso104.org/parents/nutrition.html
The website of the American Youth Soccer Organization has a section on nutrition tips for young athletes.

http://www.gssiweb.com/
The Gatorade Sports Science Institute's website has a section in their Sports Science Laboratory dedicated to youth in sports.

http://www.aces.edu/pubs/docs/H/HE-0750/
The Alabama A&M and Auburn University has an article on their website in the section of sports nutrition for young adults entitled *Eating Before and Between Athletic Events*.

INDEX